THE **nia** GUIDE FOR BLACK WOMEN

Choosing
Health and Wellness

EDITED BY SHERYL HUGGINS

AND

CHERYL MAYBERRY MCKISSACK

AGATE

Chicago

Also by Sheryl Huggins and Cheryl Mayberry McKissack

The Nia Guide for Black Women:
Achieving Career Success on Your Terms

The Nia Guide for Black Women:
Balancing Work and Life

———————

Library of Congress Cataloging-in-Publication Data

The nia guide for black women : choosing health and wellness / edited by Sheryl Huggins and Cheryl Mayberry McKissack.
    p. cm.
    Summary: "Third in a series of empowerment guides for Black women developed by the editors and contributors to NiaOnline.com. Offers practical advice for making positive choices in order to foster wellness in every aspect of life with tips, suggestions, and personal stories from successful Black women. Includes a list of resources specifically for women of color"—Provided by publisher.
    Includes bibliographical references and index.
    ISBN 1-932841-06-7 (pbk. : alk. paper)
    1. African American women—Health and hygiene. I. Huggins, Sheryl. II. McKissack, Cheryl Mayberry.

    RA778.4.A36N53 2005
    613'.04244'08996073—dc22

                                                                    2005017010

10 9 8 7 6 5 4 3 2 1

This book and all the books in *The Nia Guide for Black Women* series are available in bulk at discount prices. For more information, go to www.niaonline.com or agatepublishing.com.

This book is designed to provide accurate, authoritative information regarding its subject matter. However, it is sold with the understanding that neither the editors, authors, or publisher are medical professionals, and they are not engaged in the provision of medical advice or services. This book is not intended to be a substitute for obtaining competent medical advice; if such advice is required, the services of a competent medical professional should be obtained.

Contents

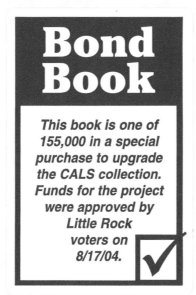

DEDICATION

From Cheryl: To my dear friend Rhonda: You are my role model for showing all of us how in the face of adversity, you have elected to choose health and wellness every day. We are so lucky to have you touch our lives through your indomitable spirit, your warm heart, and the beauty of your being. To my precious brother Brett: Life has given you many health challenges and you continue to face them every day. I am so proud of you and so lucky to have you as my brother.

From Sheryl: To my mother Angela: I have watched you face down mortality more than once, and come back better than ever. Thank you for choosing to fight life's most important battle with continual courage and grace. My own choice is to live by your example.

INTRODUCTION &
ACKNOWLEDGEMENTS

Remember that television commercial for the cholesterol-lowering drug where the handsome, fit-looking, middle-aged man struts toward a swimming pool to the strains of bossa-nova music? He looks around at the young women admiring him and flexes his muscles. As he dives in, the screen reads, "Cholesterol: 258," after which his belly-flop landing splashes the young hotties and displaces most of the water in the pool. The message is: just because you look good on the outside, doesn't mean you are healthy on the inside.

It's a message that applies to many black women. We take care of business when it comes to fashion and good grooming. In fact, in a 2004 survey of NiaOnline's Consumer Advisory Panel, grooming and appearance ranked near the bottom of the list of things that black women said they were most willing to sacrifice in their daily lives. Guess what was at the top? Exercise. Good nutrition was ranked number three, after household chores.

Black women's priorities are reflected in the fact that more then two-thirds of us are classified as overweight or obese, yet nearly half report not having any form of regular physical activity (more than a few are afraid of sweating out their hairdos, we suspect). Our priorities are also reflected in the fact that heart disease—for which obesity is a contributing factor—kills African American women at four times the rate of white women.

We could go on and on with statistics about the poor state of African American women's health in comparison to other groups (and you will encounter many more such numbers in this book), but we haven't created this book to bury you in faceless statistics, or even to make you feel bad. Instead we, the edi-tors of NiaOnline (www.niaonline.com), have created *Choosing Health and Wellness* to help black women better understand what's really going on inside of them health-wise, and what choices we face if we wish to live healthy, happy, and productive lives.

The most important of these choices is to make your good health and wellness a priority, and accept that it takes work to maintain. As co-editor of this book Cheryl Mayberry McKissack says in her chapter "The Challenge of the Forties: Making Wellness a Priority," "Choosing wellness means acknowledging that wellness is not just given to us and that, even though there is no guarantee that we will remain healthy, there are steps all of us can take to assist the process." She goes on to say, "Choosing wellness means accepting that none of the success that any of us will achieve will be greater than enjoying wellness and good health. Wellness is the essential ingredient in our enjoyment of the success that we strive to achieve. Without a healthy body, mind, and spirit, nothing else matters."

In the first book of The Nia Guide for Black Women series, we focused on how you could "achieve career success on your terms." In the second one, we addressed how to "balance work and life." This latest book in the series addresses the foundation without which those other pursuits aren't even possible: good health and wellness.

Among the topics addressed in *Choosing Health and Wellness* are:

- What are the top health issues that black women face?
- How do our race and gender affect our health?
- How do we find the time to pursue better health when there are so many demands on our time?
- What are some simple ways to incorporate better health into our daily routines?
- How can we achieve greater peace of mind?
- Where can we go for help with our health-related questions?
- How can better health habits translate into greater beauty on the outside?

You will also find examples of how famous women, such as comedian Mo'Nique and singer Lalah Hathaway, are choosing health and wellness in their own lives. Finally, three members of the Nia Guide team, co-editors Sheryl Huggins and Cheryl Mayberry McKissack, and NiaOnline communications manager Jessica Willis, share their own stories of how they are pursuing better health as black women in their twenties, thirties, and forties.

About NiaOnline and The Nia Guide Team

Since October 2000, as the web's premiere resource for, by, and about black women and their families, NiaOnline has shared expert advice about balancing work and life and finding your purpose (nia means "purpose" in Swahili). Through our annual

Nia Enterprises Leadership Summit Series, we have connected the top sisters in their fields with women who are eager succeed and grow. Through our online Consumer Advisory Panel, which reaches over 125,000 black women and their families, we have been privy to the personal views of black women. *The Nia Guide for Black Women: Choosing Health and Wellness* pulls all of this wisdom together. We hope you will enjoy reading it as much as we enjoyed putting it together.

The Nia Guide for Black Women: Choosing Health and Wellness is the latest leg of a journey begun by Cheryl Mayberry McKissack, who is the founder, president, and CEO of Nia Enterprises. Her co-editor, Sheryl E. Huggins, is editor-in-chief of NiaOnline and vice president of information services of Nia Enterprises. In addition, Jessica Willis has also contributed considerable effort in helping to assemble the Resource Guide in the back of the book.

Black Women's Health Imperative, the Washington, D.C.–based nonprofit organization devoted to improving the health of America's black women and girls, has made an enormous contribution to this book. Many thanks are due to its president and CEO, Dr. Lorraine Cole, as well as its director of membership and affiliate relations, Ingrid Padgett.

Also contributing to the book and its various constituent elements are Nia Enterprises' vice president of sales and marketing, Heather Davis; vice president and chief technology officer, Darcy Prather; and office manager and assistant to the CEO, Yvette Shelby.

As always, our heartfelt thanks to publisher of this book series, Doug Seibold, president of Agate Publishing in Chicago. We also thank project editor Patrick Lohier for the many hours he has put into *Choosing Health and Wellness*, as well as Nick Soper and the rest of the Agate team. Editor Teresa Ridley also deserves recognition for the time she put into shaping the book into final form. Kudos go to NiaOnline's health writer, Hilary Beard, for her exemplary coverage of black women's health issues over the years.

We also thank other writers who contributed to material from which this book is adapted, including, but not limited to: Carolyn Brown, Ayana Byrd, Dr. Jeff Gardere, Dorothy Randall Gray, Sherri McGee, and Allison Abner.

PART 1

BETTER HEALTH:

WHAT CHOICE DO WE HAVE?

The Black Women's Health Imperative

on the STATE OF BLACK

WOMEN'S HEALTH

Since its creation in 1983, the Black Women's Health Imperative, formerly the National Black Women's Health Project, has been devoted to improving the health of America's 19.3 million black women and girls—physically, mentally, and spiritually. Founded by health activist Byllye Y. Avery, the Washington DC–based nonprofit organization has also been a pioneer in promoting the empowerment of African American women as educated health-care consumers. So when NiaOnline decided to do Choosing Health and Wellness, *getting Black Women's Health Imperative's input was a no-brainer. We asked the organization to contribute two chapters of this book: this one and "Walking for Wellness." In this chapter, Black Women's Health*

Imperative's president and CEO, Lorraine Cole, Ph.D., provides an overview of the current state of black women's health and what we can do to improve it.

How do black women fare, health-wise, in comparison with the general population? Most people are surprised to learn that compared with other groups of women in the United States, black women have the worst health status [as measured by] nearly all of the major health indices. When it comes to chronic diseases, black women have the highest rate of hypertension, diabetes, stroke, arthritis, and lupus. When it comes to mortality, black women have the highest rate of death from heart disease, lung cancer, breast cancer, stroke, AIDS, and even pregnancy. When it comes to longevity, black women have the shortest life expectancy. Despite this devastating health portrait, there is no national sense of urgency about these startling facts. The issue of black women's health often gets lost in the larger discussions of minority health and women's health in general.

Why is the state of black women's health so poor? Numerous explanations have been published in the medical and public-health literature to account for the tremendous health divide that separates black women from nearly every other group. The most frequent explanations relate to lifestyle issues, diet, and lack of access to high-quality health care. While these are all certainly key factors, there are other factors that appear less often in print and are rarely talked about out loud. Disproportionately, black women:

- Lack adequate health-insurance coverage
- Receive the poorest quality of care, even with health insurance

3

- Have limited access to health information, new technologies, and the full range of health-care options
- Encounter an interaction of racism and sexism within the health-care system
- Have too few culturally competent health-care providers from which to choose

According to the Institute of Medicine report *Unequal Treatment*, racial disparities in medical treatment can be due to factors within the health-care system, factors associated with the health provider or associated with the patient, or a combination of any of these. Additionally, there isn't enough government or community support for race- and gender-specific clinical research into conditions that disproportionately affect black women.

What is the biggest health problem that black women face today?
Heart disease is the number one killer of all American women. But it kills African American women at four times the rate of white women. Each year, more than 40,000 black women die from heart disease, the causes of which are largely preventable. Risk factors for heart disease include cigarette smoking, hypertension, high blood cholesterol, obesity, physical inactivity, and diabetes. The more risk factors an individual has, the more likely it is that he or she will develop cardiovascular disease. Therefore, heart disease would certainly qualify as the biggest health problem that black women face.

Just as great a concern is the rapid spread of HIV infection among black women. Since the beginning of the HIV/AIDS epidemic in this country more than two decades ago, the disease burden has been steadily shifting from white males, predominantly in the gay community, to black females. AIDS now ranks as the number one killer of black women ages twenty-five to thirty-four. These are women in their prime reproductive years, which means that this epidemic is affecting two generations at once. Most of these women contracted the virus in their teens and early twenties.

However, older women are not escaping this epidemic. The number of AIDS cases in older women, regardless of race, is on the rise. In the last decade, AIDS cases in women over age 50 were reported to have tripled, and over half of these cases are in black and Hispanic women. Even though, in absolute numbers, more black men have AIDS than black women do, the absolute numbers for black women are rising at a staggering rate. Black women are the fastest-growing population of new cases, accounting for two-thirds (67 percent) of new AIDS cases among women. The rate of AIDS diagnoses for African American women is twenty-five times the rate for white women. By contrast, the rate of AIDS diagnoses for African American men is eight times the rate of white men.

What is your biggest health concern?

1. **Weight**	**(34.4%)**
2. **Diet/Nutrition**	**(17.1%)**
3. **Stress**	**(14.0%)**
4. **Fitness**	**(10.1%)**
5. **Illness**	**(7.8%)**
6. **Spiritual Health**	**(7.3%)**
7. **Mental Health**	**(3.8%)**
8. **None**	**(3.0%)**
9. **Sexual Health**	**(2.6%)**

Data drawn from a total of 924 respondents.

Results of the Black Women's Health Survey 2003 conducted by NiaOnline in conjunction with Black Women's Health Imperative. Ninety-nine percent of respondents were African American women ages 18 and above. Seventy percent were members of NiaOnline's Consumer Advisory Panel who took it online; the remainder were NiaOnline members who took the survey in person.

Do black women really have a weight problem? If so, why? And what are the most important steps that we can take to address it?
Yes, nearly 70 percent of black women are classified as either overweight or obese, and this trend—along with high levels of

obesity among American adults—shows no sign of reversing. Many obesity-related diseases, including diabetes, hypertension, cancer, and heart disease, are found in higher rates among African American women.

The two most important steps we can take to address weight are, first, to think of a fork as a lethal weapon and, second, to get up and move. In addition to all we know about the importance of eating low-fat, low-sugar, low-sodium, high-fiber, and "colorful" (fruits and vegetables and other) food, the size of each portion of food is key to controlling weight and maintaining health. As a general guide, an entire meal should fit neatly within the circle of a nine-inch plate, with enough space between each portion to see the plate. Most people have difficulty calculating their food content in terms of grams and calories. But if you keep in mind that every 3,500 calories creates one new pound, you are more likely to limit your calories to those that are nutrient-rich rather than empty.

Overall, 49 out of every 100 black women report that they do not do any form of regular physical activity. It is this fact that prompted the Black Women's Health Imperative to create programs that help black women move from "sedentary to something" in terms of their overall levels of physical activity. One of our signature programs, "Walking for Wellness," focuses on walking as a form of moderate physical activity (that program is described in detail in Chapter 26). It is the simplest, least expensive, and most effective type of activity for almost all women. We encourage black women to work their way up to at least 10,000 steps a day (wearing a pedometer to count steps) or to walk 30 minutes a day most days of the week. Short walks that total 30 minutes (say, three 10-minute walks) are just as effective as one 30-minute walk.

How common is fatigue among black women? How often do you hear black women say that they are tired or burned out, and how does this kind of stress affect our health? Fatigue can have so many causes, and it can be a symptom associated with a number of health conditions. It is one of the top ten health complaints of women. Fatigue occurs when we do not get enough of the things that are good for us: not enough sleep, not enough physical activity, not enough water, and not enough balance in our lives. It also occurs when we have too much of the things that are bad for us: too much sugar, too much caffeine, too much alcohol, and too much stress.

Fatigue is one of the key symptoms of clinical depression, and a disproportionately high percentage of black women report signs of depression. Depression rates are highest for working women who are also dealing with childcare or elder care. Fatigue can also be a symptom of many physical illnesses. In a recent study of women who'd suffered a heart attack, 70 percent reported that they experienced fatigue about a month before their heart attack occurred. Fatigue is associated with bacterial and viral infections, dietary deficiencies such as anemia, certain conditions such as pregnancy, the loss of iron during menstruation, and chronic diseases such as certain cancers. Fatigue can also be brought on by certain medications and medical-treatment regimens, as well as drug abuse and excessive alcohol use. In addition to being a symptom of various health

Top 3 health conditions black women told NiaOnline they had:

(Ranked in descending order)

1. **Hypertension**

2. **Depression**

3. **Asthma**

Data drawn from a total of 487 respondents.

Results of the Black Women's Health Survey 2003 conducted by NiaOnline in conjunction with Black Women's Health Imperative. Ninety-nine percent of respondents were African American women ages 18 and above. Seventy percent were members of NiaOnline's Consumer Advisory Panel who took it online; the remainder were NiaOnline members who took the survey in person.

problems, prolonged, debilitating fatigue is its own disease, known clinically as chronic fatigue syndrome (CFS).

Controlling stress requires controlling the things that are within your control. But it also requires controlling the way you respond to the things that are out of your control. Say "no" more often and try to be guilt-free about it. Remember that, try as you might, you just may not be able to do it all. Start delegating some of your responsibilities. No, they may not [be done] the same way or as well as you would [do them]. But you know that, so resist the temptation to do the work over. If you are a perfectionist, lower your standards a little. When you cannot control the situation, control your response. For instance, it really works to slowly count to ten before you respond when you are angry. Also, let go of old emotional "stuff." Forgiving can be liberating to you as well as to the person being forgiven. Don't obsess over what might have been. You cannot go back and undo things. Seek out a qualified mental-health professional, minister, or support group when you are experiencing very troubling times.

What are the three most important things that black women can do to improve their general health? There are three things that every black woman *must* do—starting now—to make a positive difference in her general health. First, take your health seriously. Commit today to taking care of your own health needs— physically, mentally, and spiritually. The majority of black women know the basic dos and don'ts of good health. But even with the best conditions, many of us delay our own care. We get too busy with jobs, deadlines, childcare, eldercare. Put yourself on your to-do list. Treat your body at least as well as you treat your car. Give it the right kind of fuel, keep the fluid levels high, check under the hood on a regular basis, and find a mechanic you trust. Always practice safety and never take the risk of a reckless joyride.

Second, raise your health IQ. Unless you are a health professional, the sum total of your formal health education was probably in some sort of school health class. But increasing your personal health knowledge deserves your lifelong commitment and calls for you to be an overachiever. No, you don't need to enroll in medical school. But you can create your own mini-medical-school experience from the wealth of information that surrounds you daily. For instance, read the health section of the newspaper, and watch the health segments of daily news programs. Search out the health articles in your favorite magazines. Get a good health reference book and begin to build a personal health library. The Black Women's Health Imperative has the most comprehensive, interactive health website (www.blackwomenshealth.org) designed specifically for African American women and their families. Take advantage of the wealth of health resources at this award-winning website.

Third, become a health activist. Advocate for yourself and your family every time you visit your health provider. Don't let her or him leave the room until all of your questions are answered (even if you have exceeded the customary time limit). Make sure you understand all of the treatment options available to you for your situation. Even if you don't have a pressing question, ask something anyway just for the opportunity to learn from an expert.

Beyond your personal circumstance, you can help to influence policy decisions that affect health matters by working through women's groups, churches, or health-advocacy organizations, such as the Black Women's Health Imperative. Good health is a human right, not a privilege. It should be a birthright of being an American. Like other human rights, health is affected by external political forces as well as by personal lifestyle and genetics. Our political institutions have an obligation to remove barriers to race and gender equity when it comes to health. Together, black women can have a resounding voice on such issues as access to health care, representation of black women in research, negative target marketing of unhealthy products in our communities, race and gender profiling in the health-care system, the shifting burden of certain diseases to black women, and many other health-policy issues. There has never been a more critical time for black women, and the men who love them, to be vigilant about ensuring that racial and gender health equity is elevated as a national priority.

2

Recognizing *and* **Preventing Diabetes**

Although three million African Americans suffer from diabetes, a frequently debilitating disease, one million of us don't know it yet because the condition is often symptom-free. Could your body be deteriorating silently? This chapter answers some basic questions regarding this disease.

Q: What is diabetes?

A: Diabetes is a hereditary metabolic disease in which the body either does not produce the hormone insulin—which cells need to convert sugar (glucose) in the bloodstream into energy—or doesn't use it properly. As a result, this glucose isn't metabolized and builds up to toxic levels.

In the black community, we often call diabetes "sugar"

or say we "have a touch of sugar," as if it were a casual and harmless condition. But even though diabetes is common—13 percent of African Americans have it, nearly two times the rate of whites—it can be life-threatening.

Contrary to popular belief, ingesting too much sugar does not, in and of itself, cause diabetes. However, ingesting too much sugar can lead to being overweight—a risk factor for diabetes. Furthermore, those who do have diabetes should cut back on sugar, which can make the disease worse.

Q: What are the possible complications of diabetes?

A: Having diabetes increases your chances of developing heart disease two- to four-fold. In fact, almost two-thirds of people who have high blood pressure have diabetes, and 65 percent of people with diabetes die of heart attack or stroke.

The disease also causes kidney disease and failure, resulting in the need for dialysis or transplants. Diabetes can lead to nerve damage, amputations, cataracts, glaucoma, and blindness.

Q: What is the difference between types of diabetes?

A: Here are the basic facts about each form of the disease:

Type 1: Formerly called juvenile- or insulin-dependent diabetes, this is actually an autoimmune condition that usually develops during childhood or adolescence but can occur anytime. In Type 1, the cells that make insulin have been destroyed, so patients take insulin shots.

Type 2: Also called adult-onset or non-insulin-dependent diabetes, it accounts for more than 90 percent of cases. In Type 2 diabetes, either the pancreas doesn't make enough insulin or the cells ignore the presence of insulin, even though the pancreas may make extra quantities to compensate.

The condition is usually triggered by obesity (when fat cells expand beyond a certain size, they seem to resist the action of insulin), according to Maudene Nelson, R.D., chair of the African American committee of the American Diabetes Association (ADA).

Prediabetes: Many people's doctors tell them that they have a "touch of diabetes." "This means that they already have diabetes," says Nelson, but it's in the earlier stages, when the body is beginning to have trouble processing sugar. Although the doctor may suggest "keeping an eye on it," for most people, excess glucose destroys the pancreas. It also damages many other organs—including arteries, kidneys, and eyes—within 10 years, leaving sufferers vulnerable to the devastating consequences of Type 2 disease.

But instead of waiting helplessly while your body collapses, use this time to make the lifestyle changes described under "Can I prevent diabetes?" below so that you can slow the progress of the disease—or even stop it in its tracks.

Q: How do I know if I'm at risk for diabetes?

A: If someone in your family has Type 2 diabetes, you're probably also genetically predisposed, but lifestyle choices can cause the genes to activate—or not.

Your risk is greater if you have a body mass index (BMI) of 25 or higher or if you are sedentary and middle-aged (over age 30 if you have a family history of the disease or are overweight; otherwise, over age 45). Another risk factor is a history of gestational diabetes. Take the ADA's free online diabetes risk test at Diabetes.org for more information.

Q: Can I prevent diabetes?

A: Taking the following steps can head off diabetes or slow its progress, which is especially important if you're prediabetic:

Screen: The American College of Endocrinology suggests that people with a family history of diabetes begin to get tested at age 30—when there's still time to make lifestyle changes that can stave off the condition—not at age 45, as other sources recommend. You should also get screened if you're over age 30 and your BMI is 25 or more, especially if you're sedentary, according to Nelson. So be sure to be assertive and ask your doctor for the test.

Exercise: You can also lower your risk of diabetes by exercising for 30 minutes, five times per week, and by managing your weight. Try adding a half-hour walk to your daily routine before work or after lunch or dinner.

Lose weight: Losing as little as 5 percent to 10 percent of your body weight lowers your risk if your BMI is 25 or greater. You'll find a BMI chart in Chapter 28, titled "Are You the Right Weight?" But instead of counting calories or following a diet, try reapportioning your plate, Nelson advises. She suggests making 50 percent of your plate vegetables; 25 percent starchy food, such as sweet potatoes, beans, and corn; and 25 percent protein, such as meat, poultry, and fish.

Because of their high vitamin, protein, and fiber content, Nelson recommends eating plenty of beans (including red, black, and lima varieties), peas (such as green, black-eyed, and pigeon peas), and lentils. It's best to avoid fried foods because the grease (trans fats) in those foods is so dangerous.

Q: What are the signs of diabetes?

A: The symptoms of the disease include the following:

- Frequent urination
- Excessive thirst
- Extreme hunger
- Unusual weight loss
- Increased fatigue
- Irritability
- Blurry vision

For more information about preventing or controlling diabetes, visit the ADA's website at Diabetes.org.

"One of the signs of insulin resistance is very dark pigmentation on the neck, armpits, and groin," says Nelson. Chronic yeast and urinary-tract infections may also signal diabetes. For more about diabetes and women, read *Women and Diabetes* by Laurinda M. Poirier (ADA; $15).

If you have any of these signs, contact your doctor immediately—but realize that one-third of sufferers have no warning at all.

Q: Why this epidemic?

A: There is a theory that people whose ancestors survived food shortages and periods of famine—including African Americans—have a "thrifty" gene that holds on to excess calories to protect them from future starvation, suggests Nelson. Now that life is more sedentary and food is overly abundant, perhaps these people are more likely to gain excess weight.

Q: What if I already have diabetes?

A: The good news about diabetes is that many people are able to manage it by following the prevention tips above— exercising, losing weight, following simple eating habits to control blood sugar levels, and, if necessary, taking proper medication. You should also know that:

- Controlling your blood pressure can reduce your risk of heart attack and stroke by 33-50 percent
- By controlling your cholesterol and triglycerides (a blood fat) you can reduce your risk of cardiovascular complications by 20-50 percent
- For every one point reduction you make in your A1C (2-3 month blood glucose trend) level, you reduce your risk of eye complications by up to 40 percent.

PART 2

STARTING WITH THE BASICS

3

The Challenge *of the* Twenties:

DEVELOPING GOOD HABITS TO LAST A LIFETIME

As a child of the South, Jessica Nyel Willis, NiaOnline's 25-year-old communications manager, knows all too well how difficult it can be to overcome a tradition of unhealthy eating and a sedentary lifestyle. But "sedentary" certainly doesn't describe Willis's career. It's her passion for media that took her from Augusta, Georgia, to New York City. She majored in telecommunications as an undergraduate at Purdue University in Indiana (her college internships included The Oprah Winfrey Show in Chicago and America's Black Forum in Washington DC). In addition to working full-time at NiaOnline, Willis has been pursuing an MBA in media management at Metropolitan College of New

York. She is also an actress and a writer of novels, short stories, magazine articles, and television scripts. In the community, Willis volunteers her time as a mentor for Imentor.org, serves as director of membership services for the Black Fashion Designers Association, and volunteers for the YB Literary Foundation. Here, she describes her own often-uncomfortable relationship with diet and exercise, as well as the healthy, sensible changes she's making to build her own legacy of wellness.

Trying to achieve a healthy lifestyle has been an interesting journey for me, one that is deeply affected by my having grown up in the South. We weren't overly concerned about healthy eating or exercising in my childhood home in Georgia. We ate and played as we wanted. Today, in my mid-twenties, I find it an ongoing challenge to balance work and graduate school with a healthy diet and a viable exercise routine. I am hoping, however, that by eating better and increasing my activity level, I will not only feel better and think faster but will also set myself on the path to a lifetime of wellness. I have seen the damaging effects of traditional Southern cooking and minimal exercise on the bodies of my mother, my aunts, and my grandmothers. The weekly phone calls from my mother (who is not even 50) about her high blood pressure and high cholesterol have only pushed me to work harder at getting my own act together.

Before embarking on improving my lifestyle, though, I decided to learn more about the role that a legacy of Southern cooking and exercise aversion had played in my life.

Bad Habits Start Early

Being from the South, I was never one to shy away from food. I used to be that skinny girl who ate like a horse and whose dinner plate was almost as big as her father's. I felt as if I won a trophy every time someone commented on how much I ate but never gained an ounce. Although I grew up in the fast-food era, my parents cooked a lot. To this day, my favorite meal is still my mother's fried chicken, homemade mashed potatoes, collard greens, and corn bread with a cola on the side.

Exercise encouragement in my house consisted of, "Go outside and play. Get some sun." I was a precocious child and often preferred reading a book in my room to playing games outdoors. I never liked that "outside" smell you got after playing in the grass for several hours. When my brother and I were older, we joined recreational softball and baseball teams, but that was the extent of my forays into sports or exercise. I remember that I did play tennis for one semester of high school, but I wasn't very good and soon quit.

Once I got to college, at Purdue University in Lafayette, Indiana, I was still a long (I've been five feet eight since ninth grade) and lean size eight. For the first two years, I ate in the dorm and never missed a meal. My junior year, I moved into a dorm apartment and started cooking my own food—or ate fast food. Snacking at night while I was studying or at a group meeting was a normal occurrence. I drank lots of soda, Kool-Aid, and fruit juice and was, in fact, lucky if I drank one cup of water a day. I did not exercise, even though a huge recreational facility was available to all students and faculty for free. I can count on both hands the number of times I actually stepped foot inside the "co-rec." Still, by the time I finished college, I had gained only five pounds.

The years since then, however, have brought changes. I had prided myself on never gaining that "freshman 15," but at age 25, I found those words beginning to haunt me. The extra 15 pounds had finally caught up with me, and I noticed that my energy level was substantially lower. I liked to think that I could blame some of these changes on simply being older, but not all of them. I had never cultivated the habits of eating healthfully and exercising. Looking at myself in the mirror and feeling my body's sluggishness, I seriously began to reconsider my approach to health and wellness.

A Shared, Unhealthy Legacy

When I began to reflect on my attitudes toward food and exercise and wonder about their origins, I didn't have to look far beyond my Southern heritage. I truly believe that one of the legacies of slavery is the culture of unhealthy eating. According to Joseph E. Holloway, Ph.D., who wrote the article "African Crops and Slave Cuisine" for Slaveryinamerica.org, our slave ancestors were forced to eat the less savory and less healthy portions of the pig or cow. Fatty portions of the animal, like ham hocks, neck bones, pig feet, and chitlins, were common servings on a slave's plate. To compensate for the poor quality of the meat, the slaves often added a lot of salt and fat. Fried chicken was also a staple because chickens were abundant and easy to divide up to feed many mouths. After our ancestors were freed, they continued to prepare and eat the foods that they had become accustomed to and now loved. They ate the meals that their grandmothers had prepared and their mothers had prepared before them.

In addition to a bad diet, particularly in the South, too many of us have just not embraced exercising. During slavery, black people stayed fit by toiling all day in the fields. But as our fore-fathers and foremothers made the transition from the fields to factories, and from stores to offices, the labor became less intensive. African Americans have gradually gotten heavier, most notably because our diets have not changed dramatically. But let's face it: When faced with the choice between exercise and leisure, most of us have tended to opt for leisure.

Southerners are also faced with intense summer heat. When the temperature reaches 100-plus degrees across those South-ern states, it is suicide to attempt to exercise outdoors. So the prevailing attitude becomes, if you want to exercise, you have to join a gym. But if joining a gym is too expensive, then you just don't do anything. These observations are in no way meant to stereotype all black people from the South, but they are a true representation of what I have witnessed in my own up-bringing and family.

Forging a New Relationship With Exercise

Analyzing and understanding this legacy was one thing, but coming up with a solution to enhance my own wellness was a whole other story. My first approach was to tackle the lack of physical activity in my life. I work in front of a computer for eight hours a day and then spend even more time at the com-puter completing assignments for graduate school, working on my next novel, and tackling projects for community organiza-tions. Suffice it to say that I spend at least 10 to 12 hours per day sitting in front of a computer. It's not surprising that my sed-entary lifestyle was taking a toll on my body.

About six months after graduating from college, I bought a couple of Tae-Bo tapes and attempted to work out to them at least two or three mornings per week. I did this off and on for several months and then gave up. I bought a Tony Little Gazelle

Freestyle exercise machine and used it two or three times a week for several months, but I gave that up too. I then joined the Lucille Roberts gym, signing a two-year contract. I went at least a few times a month for about a year, upped my attendance to at least twice per week for several months, and then quit altogether with a few months left on my contract. I had become frustrated by the system in place at my particular gym that allowed women to reserve machines for their friends, even when their friends weren't there.

Out of all those stops and starts and stops again, I did learn a few things about my relationship with working out: I find exercise boring, and I do not like to sweat. I do, however, like to work out in the morning, and I like to do it to hip-hop music because I can sing or rap along with the artists, taking my mind off the tediousness of the activity and the sweat dripping down my back.

Still, when I added graduate studies to my full-time work schedule last fall, I pushed exercise to the side once again, using the excuse that I did not have enough time. Once winter arrived, I decided that it was too cold outside to exercise, not even considering working out indoors. With the arrival of spring, though, I resolved to start again. I recently bought an MP3 player so that I can listen to hip-hop as I run. I also took the next step to wellness: I went jogging by myself. Over the last three weeks, I've gone jogging four times.

As a novice runner, I am thrilled that I have accomplished such a feat, and not under threat of violence. My goal is to build up to three times per week, but that will come one week at a time. Right now I am working on two times a week, four weeks in a row. I've also used the resources of the MSN Health and Fitness network (www.health.msn.com/fitness) to learn about exercises and stretches that I can do at home if the weather is bad or if I don't feel like running. Sure, things will happen to throw me off schedule, as they have in the past, but what's important is for me to get up out of bed and back on track.

A Sensible Diet Plan You Can Live With

During my exercise experiments, I began to look at different established diets that would train me to eat well and help me to lose weight. After careful research, I settled on the South Beach Diet. I can hear your groans—"Not another diet"—but this eating plan truly helped me to understand my body, the food I eat, and how that food affects my body. According to Arthur S. Agatston, MD, creator of the South Beach Diet, the basic premise of the plan is not to think about eating low-carb or low-fat but to eat the right carbs and the right fats. I actually lost seven pounds in two weeks on the diet.

Even though I no longer believe that a specific diet plan is the route to go, because it is not something I can feasibly maintain over a lifetime, I have incorporated several things from the South Beach Diet into what I simply call eating healthy. This isn't about bean sprouts and tofu (although both are very good); it's about practical tips that you can gradually apply to help you lose weight and give your body the boost it needs. These tips include the following:

Drink more water. You have to drink water to hydrate and cleanse the body. People are often intimidated by the thought of having to drink so many ounces per day. I suggest using a visual cue instead. I learned that I drink more water from a bottle than I do from a glass. I selected a 16-ounce bottle with a pleasing shape and feel (both important things), and I fill it up and drink the contents at least three times per day. Although three bottles do not add up to the 64 ounces a day that some experts recommend, they get pretty close, and the total is still a lot more water than I've ever drunk at any other time in my life.

Eat multiple meals a day. You can't skip meals. If you do, you'll wind up ravenous and eat more calories in one meal than you would have in two. You must eat, at the very minimum, breakfast, lunch, and dinner. If you don't eat at least three squares a day now, get up in the morning and train yourself. Even if it's just with a bagel and cream cheese, you have to jump-start your metabolism for the day so that you can burn calories faster. Some experts even suggest eating five meals per day. (The South Beach Diet recommends three meals a day, plus two snacks if you get hungry.) Do whatever works for you; just be sure to watch your portions. Eat slowly, and when you're full, walk away. We are trained as kids to clean our plates, but this is a very bad thing to do. If you are no longer hungry, that means your body is satisfied and you should stop eating.

Reduce the amount of bread and rice in your diet. We are raised with the notion that no meal is complete without a meat, a vegetable, and usually two starches (such as potatoes and bread). The South Beach Diet cautions you to limit the amount of starches in your diet, particularly bread and rice. I've learned to enjoy a meat with two vegetables and no starch, especially not processed white bread or white rice. I recently asked my grandmother for a bread maker for Christmas so that I can bake fresh, whole-grain bread that is healthier than store-bought wheat bread. I'm not saying never eat bread or rice; I'm saying, everything in moderation.

Lighten up on the salt. Salt makes just about everything taste better, but too much of it can also contribute to heart disease and high blood pressure. Incorporate other herbs and spices into your diet, and use less salt. Try fresh herbs like garlic, dill, and cilantro, which can add unique flavors.

Cut down on fat. Eat lean meats. Use all-vegetable oil or olive oil, not the leftover bacon grease from breakfast. Don't slather on the butter, and consider using margarine or reduced-fat butter instead. Try to move from whole milk to two-percent or even one-percent milk. And consider choosing low-fat or reduced-fat cheese.

A Journey of a Lifetime

By incorporating these small changes in my diet, as well as exercising twice a week, I have noticed a significant change in my body. My skin is much healthier-looking—it's more even-toned, and I have fewer blemishes. I feel more energetic and don't hit the snooze button as often in the morning. My breathing is better, and I have fewer stress headaches than before. I'm more even-tempered and happier than I've been in months.

This is an ongoing process, and it has not been easy. There are days and sometimes weeks of relapses, but after goading myself a bit, I get back on track. Always remember that you can start over again tomorrow. Just don't let that become your never-ending mantra. For me, it's not about fitting back into those slim-fit jeans or wearing a midriff-baring top during the summer (which I've never done anyway). It is not about denying myself, either. I occasionally treat myself to a hamburger and fries, or brownies with vanilla ice cream and a tall glass of whole milk. But I recognize the consequences of eating such things, and I know that I cannot eat them on a regular basis.

My goal is to learn and practice habits of wellness now that will serve me for the rest of my life. When I get to be my mother's age and my grandmother's age, I want to be fit and as free from illness as possible. But in addition, I want to build a foundation for the children I plan to have. I want to instill in them the importance of watching what you eat and how much you eat, and treating your body well. I've got a long way to go, but I know it will be a wonderful journey.

4

HOW TO GET
the Sleep You Need

If you're like most women, you sleep an average of seven hours or less a night. For those of us bringing home work, helping the kids with their homework, doing the laundry, and fixing dinner—all while trying to squeeze in a little time for ourselves—seven hours, or even six, may seem like a luxury. To make matters worse, up to 60 percent of Americans suffer from symptoms of insomnia.

But sleeplessness takes its toll: Long-term sleep loss results in low-grade depression, among other problems. So you owe it to yourself to make sure you're getting the sleep you need. Experts say that we need eight hours. Here are some ways for you to catch up on your Z's:

Exercise: Getting about 20 to 30 minutes of exercise daily helps relieve stress and anxiety that can keep you awake. But be sure to exercise several hours before going to sleep, since exercise can also keep you alert.

Make love: Sex, which is really a form of moderate exercise, can help you fall asleep. There are those of us, however, who are energized by sex. If that describes you, schedule sex well before bedtime.

Don't try to sleep: Trying to sleep—and obsessing over how you can't fall asleep—makes it harder for you to sleep. Let sleep take you over by reading, listening to relaxing music, or meditating until you're drowsy.

Limit caffeine and eliminate nicotine: Both substances are stimulants that can keep you awake. Cut down to no more than two cups of coffee—drunk before noon. And of course, quit smoking.

Sleep in bed: Sounds silly, but many of us use our beds as one big desk, table, and recliner all in one. We do everything from reading and eating to watching TV, writing, and talking on the phone. Limit your bedroom to sleep (and sex, of course).

Check your meds: Some medications may be preventing you from sleeping. Many prescription and over-the-counter (OTC) drugs such as cold remedies and painkillers contain caffeine and other stimulants. Read labels carefully, and ask your physician about the side effects of all prescription medication.

Be careful with alcohol: While a glass of wine can relax you, overdoing it can actually cause middle-of-the-night awakenings from dehydration. If you drink alcohol, also take in several glasses of water at least an hour before bedtime (so you don't wake up to go to the bathroom).

Keep a regular schedule: As often as you can, wake up at the same time every day. This will help you regulate your internal clock. Limit naps to 20 minutes several hours before bedtime.

Think "cool room, warm feet": As strange as it sounds, you need a cool room and warm feet to fall asleep. Keep your room at a comfortably low temperature, and wear socks if you need to.

Create a good sleeping environment: This sounds obvious, but if your room is too loud—or, for some, too quiet—add background or "white" noise. Fans, air purifiers, and even noise machines create a constant, soothing sound that drowns out distracting noises.

Talk to your doctor: If your sleeping problems persist for more than two weeks, it's time to speak to your health-care practitioner. She or he may recommend that you visit a sleep clinic; suggest an OTC supplement, such as melatonin; or prescribe temporary medication to help you with insomnia.

5

DO YOU NEED

More Sleep?

Andrea Hinton, of Detroit, hadn't slept well since she learned that her company would relocate to another city and she would lose her marketing position at the end of the year. "I toss and turn at night thinking of worst-case scenarios," says the single mother of a first-grader. "Everyone's leaving here; there aren't many jobs in my field."

Almost 60 percent of adults experience at least one symptom of insomnia several nights a week, and 35 percent have shown signs of insomnia either every night or almost every night over the past year, according to the National Sleep Foundation. Are you one of these sleep-deprived folks? Read on.

"Ms. Hinton's is clearly a very difficult life situation and a major life stressor," says Helene Emsellem, M.D., director of the Center for Sleep and Wake Disorders in Chevy Chase, Maryland. "It's not surprising that her sleep is suffering."

Hinton had insomnia, a condition whose symptoms include the following:

- Difficulty falling asleep.
- Waking up frequently during the night.
- Awaking too early and having a hard time falling asleep again.
- Waking up and not feeling refreshed.

What Causes Insomnia?

Stress: Whether school or job pressures; family, marital, or relationship problems; serious illness; or a death in the family, stress is the number one cause of a bad night's sleep. "I fall asleep OK but then wake up in the middle of the night, and my mind races until about 5 a.m.," Hinton said. "When my alarm clock goes off at 5:45, I'm already beat!"

If you wake up worrying, Dr. Emsellem recommends this approach: "During the daylight hours, set aside purposeful worrying time when you can make a list of strategies, decide how you're going to approach the problem, make up a budget, and put your anxieties on paper. This relieves the brain of having to reshuffle these thoughts all night long."

When such stressful events pass, insomnia often does too. If it doesn't, you may be experiencing low-grade depression, anxiety, or a sleep disorder. These include sleep apnea, a serious and potentially life-threatening condition, often characterized by snoring, in which brief interruptions of breathing awaken the sleeper; and restless legs syndrome, which is marked by an urge to move the legs and often includes involuntary leg twitches and kicks that can disrupt rest.

Lifestyle: If you are drinking caffeinated beverages such as coffee, tea, or soda (even clear sodas often contain caffeine) in the afternoon or evening, or eating chocolate, which is also caffeinated, you can end up staring at the ceiling at night.

Hinton occasionally enjoyed a glass of red wine. "Alcohol does have relaxing and sedating qualities, but it also disrupts the quality and quantity of sleep," says Dr. Emsellem. "Drink it as far away from bedtime as possible." The nicotine in cigarettes, which may seem to calm you down, actually stimulates you. Eating after 8:00 p.m. can also keep your eyes wide open because your digestive system's activity interferes with sleep.

Shift work: Especially if you work first or third shift, you may be trying to force yourself to snooze when the sun, your environment, and your biological rhythms are all trying to keep you awake.

Environment: Many people find it hard to zone out when there is noise outside; the TV is blaring in another room; or if their partner has different sleeping habits, is snoring, or tossing and turning right next to them.

How to Get Your Z's

If you don't nip insomnia in the bud, you may find yourself chronically unable to get to sleep and experiencing physical, mental, or emotional health problems, including difficulty concentrating, irritability, and even high blood pressure. Try implementing these steps as soon as possible:

- Remove the phone, TV, computer, and other waking-hour activities from your bedroom. Use your boudoir only for sleeping, having sex, and engaging in pleasant and soothing activities.
- Take a chill pill. Dietary supplements such as calcium (1,500 to 2,000 milligrams) and magnesium (1,000 mg)

can have a relaxing and calming effect. Take doses after meals and before bedtime.

- If you're a night owl trying to live in a 9-to-5 world, taking .5 mg of the dietary supplement melatonin 8 to 10 hours after your weekday wake-up time (not at bedtime) can reset your sleep-wake cycle. "Taking it late at night as a sleeping pill can actually delay the onset of sleep," Dr. Emsellem says.
- Two hours before bedtime, remove as many sources of stress from your environment as possible. Put your family on notice that you're taking "me" time, Dr. Emsellem recommends. Draw a hot bath, stretch gently, read, or enjoy soft music.
- According to *Prescription for Nutritional Healing* (Avery; $24), the herbs valerian, kava, and California poppy can promote relaxation. Rotate among them. A few drops of lavender, sweet orange, or chamomile oil can add fragrance to your bath and calm you.
- If it's loud on your street or if others are awake in your home, a white noise CD or machine may desensitize you to outside sounds.
- Lie flat on your back, placing your hand on your abdomen, below your navel. Deep-breathe for about 10 minutes, making your hand rise and fall. As your mind wanders, bring it back to your hand and focus on breathing again.
- Calculate the number of hours you are actually sleeping and allow yourself only that many hours in bed. Every few days, increase your scheduled sleep time by 15 minutes. "When you take away time spent lying anxious in bed, you reinforce a positive sleep experience," says Dr. Emsellem. Leave your bed and your bedroom only after

you've given yourself a reasonable amount of time to nod off, Dr. Emsellem suggests. Go into another room to read with a book light, listen to soft music, or work a crossword puzzle—but don't get wound up surfing the internet or watching TV. When you feel sleepy, return to bed.

- Over-the-counter sleep medications may help occasional problems, but "people develop a tolerance for them," says Dr. Emsellem. If insomnia persists, see your doctor. "There are better medicines to use for sleep," she says. Dr. Emsellem encourages Hinton to go on the offensive and develop practical strategies for dealing with her situation. But if she continues to awaken early, fatigue may undermine her ability to handle her challenges. "There are appropriate indications for the use of prescription sleep aids; her situation may be one," Dr. Emsellem says.

6

Go With the Flow:

THE TRUTH ABOUT WATER AND GOOD HEALTH

Anyone who has ever read a women's magazine knows that it's important to stay hydrated, not just during exercise but throughout the day. But integrating water into your life can leave you feeling tethered to the bathroom *and* a water bottle.

Exactly how much H2O do you need, though? As you've probably noticed, experts now seem to disagree, and it can be hard to get enough water without cramping your lifestyle. It can also be tough to pick among the different types of water—should you drink spring, seltzer, mineral, plain old tap? Do you really need a water purifier and, if so, how do you choose the right one? For the answers, read on.

At least two-thirds of the human body is made up of water, its most important component. Water helps digest food, dissolves nutrients so they can circulate in the bloodstream, removes waste and toxins, helps cells communicate, regulates body temperature, and lubricates moving parts.

Drinking enough water can help prevent kidney stones as well as cancers of the urinary tract and colon, according to nutritionist Goulda Downer, Ph.D., RD, of Metroplex Health and Nutrition Services in Washington DC. One study by the National Cancer Institute (NCI) found that "women who drank five or more glasses a day were 45 percent less likely to develop colon cancer than those who drank less than two glasses a day," she says.

Breathing, perspiring, and going to the bathroom cause us to lose between 6 and 12.5 cups of water each day, according to *Nutrition for Dummies* (IDG Books; $20). Replenish your supply too slowly and your gums, tongue, and teeth will dry out, causing you to feel thirsty. Your skin may dry out, and your lips may become chapped. Habitually drink too little water and you may become dehydrated. Symptoms include fatigue, lethargy, weakness, dizziness, headaches, and even sunken eyes, Dr. Downer says.

If you are drinking enough fluids to stay hydrated and healthy, your urine will be pale. (Note: Some vitamins may turn your urine bright yellow, so check the color on a day when you skip your vitamins.) "Going to the bathroom at least once in the middle of the night is also a sign of good hydration status," Dr. Downer states.

Obey Your Thirst?

But not all liquids are equally hydrating. For instance, the NCI study found that the women who drank water were less likely to develop colon cancer than women who drank other beverages, Dr. Downer explains. She suggests drinking four to six 8-ounce glasses of water each day and making sure that your total fluid intake—which may include juices, coffee, and soup, among other liquids—ranges from 64 to 80 ounces. Eating lots of fruits and veggies will also help keep you hydrated. Lettuce, for example, is about 90 percent water, while a bagel contains about 30 percent.

Why is water better than other fluids? Drinks containing natural and artificial sugars, such as juices, juice drinks, and sodas, often contain 100 or so calories per 8-ounce glass. These days, who has extra calories to spare?

Caffeinated drinks, including coffee, tea, and many sodas, provide water but also act as mild diuretics, increasing the amount of water the body eliminates. For every 8-ounce caffeinated beverage you consume, you'll need to drink 4 to 8 ounces of water to offset the fluid loss. And alcohol "has a profoundly diuretic effect," Dr. Downer says, even if you drink only beer or wine coolers.

Water, Water Everywhere . . .

Many people find that carrying bottled water is a convenient way to help them keep track of the number of ounces they've consumed.

You may choose to save money by filling your water bottle at home. Be sure to wash it daily to prevent bacteria from growing. If you drink a lot of highly seasoned, sweet, or salty foods, you may dislike water's bland taste. If so, spruce it up until your taste buds adjust to milder flavors. Try adding a zip of orange or lemon juice. Or ease your transition to plain water by incorporating flavored waters into the mix. But do so knowing this: Flavored waters are often high in calories, so drinking more than one or two a day may not be a realistic option if you're keeping an eye on your weight.

Dr. Downer offers these additional tips for going with the flow:

- Try your water cold, cool, at room temperature, and warm to see which you prefer.
- Enjoy a full glass of water immediately upon awakening and before you go to sleep (although you may not want an entire glass if you need uninterrupted sleep).
- Carry a water bottle with you, spacing your consumption throughout the day, especially between meals. You may actually stave off hunger and save a few calories, too, if you drink one full glass whenever your tummy rumbles.
- Don't forget to enjoy plenty of naturally hydrating fruits and veggies.

Which Water to Drink?

Not all water will provide you with the same health benefits, however. There are impurities and additives to consider. Do you really need to buy bottled, or is tap water safe? How do bottled waters differ? Can a purifier provide the same quality as bottled, or should you save your money? To find out the answers, read on.

The federal government regulates water quality via the U.S. Environmental Protection Agency (EPA); however, experts disagree about whether tap water is actually safe from the contaminants and pollution that local water utilities are supposed to remove.

The EPA contends that tap water is safe and provides local drinking water information for most counties in the country. But a recent survey of the drinking water of 19 major cities, performed by the National Resources Defense Council, challenges the EPA's position. According to the survey, tap water often contains contaminants such as sewage and pesticides that have washed into streams.

Many people, whether to play it safe or because their tap water doesn't taste or smell good, prefer to use a purifier at home or drink bottled water. Talk to your dentist if you pursue the latter option. Bottled water may not contain fluoride, which can help keep teeth healthy, and your dentist may suggest that you receive extra fluoride treatments.

Hitting the Bottle

Just because water comes in a bottle doesn't guarantee that it's safer than tap. Stick to brands sold by members of the International Bottled Water Association, the industry trade organization.

Once you've done that, consider your preferences—and the source:

- *Spring water* comes from an underground formation through which it flows naturally to the earth's surface.
- *Mineral water*, which originates from an underground source, naturally contains "good" minerals such as calcium, magnesium, sodium, potassium, silica, and bicarbonates.
- *Artesian well water* is typically found deeper in the earth than spring water and, therefore, *may* be more pure and contain less contamination.
- *Sparkling water* (which may also be called carbonated water) flows from an underground source; carbonation is added to it later on.
- *Purified water* has been processed to remove chlorine and other compounds. If the water's source is not listed, it is probably purified municipal drinking water.
- *Distilled water* is municipal drinking water that has been boiled to remove many, though not all, contaminants.

- *Seltzer* is considered a soft drink, not bottled water, and may contain artificial sweeteners and flavors—and, therefore, calories. It may also be called soda water or club soda.
- *Flavored water* also contains calories—sometimes as many as soda. But this product can be useful in helping you make the transition from flavored beverages to plain water. (To give plain water some flavor without the calories, add a twist of lemon or orange.)
- *Nutrient-enhanced water* can contain 125 calories per bottle, yet there's no good evidence that the ingredients work, according to the *Nutrition Action Health Letter*, published by the Center for Science in the Public Interest.

Do You Need a Purifier?

Many people use purifiers to remove contaminants and make water taste and smell better. Purifiers are also economical—they can help you cut bottled-water expenditures by 50 percent or more, even when you factor in the $300 (for parts and labor) it often costs to have the system installed, according to *Consumer Reports*. But don't forget to change the filter on schedule; bacterial contamination can be more dangerous than toxins. Here are your options:

- *Filtration pitchers* are easy to use and maintain. They don't require that you wield your wrench, but they gobble refrigerator space.
- *Faucet-mounted purifiers* are easy to install and less cumbersome than pitchers.
- *Under-the-sink filters* typically require professional installation. The cartridges last longer than those in pitchers and faucets, but changing them can be tricky.

Reverse-osmosis technology is superior for treating severe flavor and pollution problems; however, the machines filter slowly and hog space.

· *Whole-house systems*—gallon per gallon, the most cost-effective—treat water as it enters your home, allowing you to drink, cook, shower, and do laundry with purified water. They can also prolong the life of appliances in areas where drinking water contains a lot of sediment.

7

Right on Time:
ADVICE ON STAYING REGULAR

Chances are, you know that a healthy diet includes at least three meals a day. Do you know, though, how many times you're supposed to eliminate the waste from those meals? Is it three bowel movements a day? Or maybe one? And if you don't do "number two" daily, are you poisoning yourself with waste?

Perhaps because talking about the topic is so taboo, myths and misconceptions abound about what constitutes healthy bowel habits. That's why NiaOnline decided to tackle this sensitive subject: to examine exactly what it means to be "regular," as well as the common reasons that healthy people get backed up, and offer some lifestyle habits to help keep your movements coming.

What Is Regular?

Regular bowel movements are essential for removing excrement and toxins from the body. Each person's rhythm for defecating differs. "The average woman has five bowel move-ments a week," says gastroenterologist Arnold Wald, M.D., spokesperson for the American Gastroenterological Associa-tion (AGA), professor of medicine at the University of Pitts-burgh, and coauthor of a study examining the facts and fiction about constipation. "The range of normal is three per week to three per day," he says.

Everyone occasionally becomes constipated, which the AGA defines as "the infrequent and difficult passage of stool." When a person goes more than three days without a bowel movement—even fewer, for some people—feces usually harden. The result? Straining and discomfort while eliminating. Although consti-pation usually isn't serious, if you're irregular for three weeks or more, develop hemorrhoids, bleed from your anus, notice bloody streaks on your stools, or experience severe pain, it's important to seek medical assistance.

Constipation's Common Causes

There are several reasons that the movement of stool through the colon might slow. Dr. Wald cautions that each person is different, so "some of these factors may or may not apply" to everyone:

- *An unbalanced diet:* According to the AGA, a diet high in animal fats—including meats, dairy products, and eggs—and refined sugar, but low in dietary fiber, can cause blockage. Yet Dr. Wald cautions that inadequate fiber should not automatically be assumed to be the cause. "People have different requirements," he says. "One person may require 25 grams a day, and another person may be fine on 10."
- *Not consuming enough liquids:* Liquids like water and

juice increase the amount of fluid in both the colon and stool, while caffeinated drinks and alcohol are dehydrating. Recommends Dr. Wald: "Fluids are good, but don't drown yourself trying to treat constipation." Drinking eight 8-ounce glasses daily should be enough.

- *Lack of exercise:* Research shows that "couch potatoes might be more constipated. Exercise is always good," Dr. Wald says.
- *Certain medications:* These may include antacids containing aluminum and magnesium, antidepressants, blood pressure medications (calcium channel blockers), iron supplements, and some pain medications.
- *Irritable bowel syndrome (IBS):* Causing alternating constipation and diarrhea, IBS is one of constipation's most common causes. Treatments are available, so if you think you have IBS, be sure to check with your doctor.
- *Ignoring the urge:* "This is particularly common among women, who may not want to excuse themselves from activities or use public restrooms," Dr. Wald observes. Delaying bowel movements can lead to "acquired constipation," in which your body learns to become backed up, he says.
- *Abuse of laxatives:* "The myth that you have to have a bowel movement daily to be healthy has led to the misuse of laxatives," Dr. Wald says. "For a person with occasional constipation, it is safe to take a stimulant laxative one or two times a week."
- *Travel:* Lifestyle changes associated with traveling may alter your diet, drinking habits, or schedule, consequently cramping your style.
- *Hormones:* Many women complain that they become backed up during their menstrual cycle. As hormone

levels change, some, but not all, women experience constipation, according to Dr. Wald. Women are also more likely to become irregular while pregnant, when a combination of hormones and pressure on the colon makes passing stools more difficult. "Particularly late in pregnancy, there is evidence that hormones can inhibit the bowel," Dr. Wald explains.

It probably won't surprise you to learn that eating a balanced diet containing lots of fruits, vegetables, and whole grains, along with exercising regularly and drinking plenty of water, can help keep you regular. Or that indulging in a steady diet of fast food, refined (processed) products, and fried foods can keep you backed up.

But if you pigged out on fast-food french fries and burgers Saturday night anyway and now you're constipated, you're probably looking for more immediate relief—not a guilt trip.

The Truth About Laxatives

Laxatives help you go to the bathroom sooner or without straining. There are several types, stimulant laxatives being the most common. But rumors about their safety—particularly if they're used regularly—abound.

You may have heard some variation of this urban legend: If you use laxatives too often, your colon will stop working on its own, you will need larger and larger doses, and you can damage your colon or even develop colon cancer. But Dr. Wald's study shows these beliefs to be unfounded. Taken according to directions, "laxatives are quite safe and effective," Dr. Wald says.

Dr. Wald is less certain about the safety of laxative teas. They typically contain the same stimulant, senna, found in several of the major over-the-counter laxative brands, but they combine it with other ingredients. "You can vary the strength of the laxative by varying the strength of the tea," he says, making it difficult to determine the dose you are taking.

In addition, the ingredients vary and can affect people differently. Celestial Seasonings, maker of Good Nite Cleanse, notes that people with gallstones should not take it. The website of Traditional Medicinals, which makes Smooth Moves tea, provides detailed instructions on how to brew it. So if you do decide to use any of these teas, read the labels carefully and follow instructions.

Which Laxative Category Is Right for You?

Stimulant

- *How it works:* By causing the muscles of the intestine to contract and expel stools.
- *How long it takes:* From two to six hours to overnight; faster if taken on an empty stomach.
- *Word to the wise:* May cause side effects such as cramping, diarrhea, and nausea.
- *Major brands:* Dulcolax, Ex-Lax, and Senokot. Major tea brands include Smooth Moves, Good Nite Cleanse, and Get Regular by Yogi Teas.

Bulk-forming fiber supplement

- *How it works:* By absorbing water from the intestine and increasing stool bulk and softness, thus triggering the intestine to expel it.
- *How long it takes:* Typically 12 hours.
- *Word to the wise:* Drink plenty of water, or it may make you more constipated.
- *Major brands:* Citrucel, FiberCon, and Metamucil.

Stool softener (emollient)

- *How it works:* Helps to soften stools so bowels move without straining.
- *How long it takes:* One to two days.
- *Word to the wise:* Doesn't promote bowel movements.
- *Major brands:* Colace and Surfak.

Lubricant

- *How it works:* Coats the bowel and stools with a waterproof film that allows easier passage; also prevents stools from becoming hard and dry.
- *How long it takes:* Six to eight hours.
- *Word to the wise:* Blocks the absorption of some vitamins and minerals if taken two hours before or after a meal; not for long-term use; not for people who suffer from acid reflux.
- *Major brands:* Look for the generic mineral oil.

Saline

- *How it works:* Significantly increases water content of stools by drawing water to them.
- *How long it takes:* From 30 minutes to three hours—or as long as overnight.
- *Word to the wise:* Not for long-term use or repeated relief.
- *Major brands:* Look for the generic milk of magnesia or Epsom salt; directions for use as a laxative appear on the label.

Laxatives are powerful medicines, so read their labels carefully, as you would with any medicine. Exercise particular care if you're pregnant or breast-feeding or if you have high blood pressure, heart disease, diabetes, kidney disease, or an in-flamed colon.

If you find yourself needing frequent assistance with having a bowel movement, talk to your doctor about what you can do to prevent or manage your constipation.

PART 3

SEEKING SENSE AND SANCTUARY

8

ARE YOU

Depressed?

Would your friends and family describe you as "a downer"? Do you find the negative in every situation? Are you generally dissatisfied with your life? Do you feel low most of the time and have little energy?

If you answered yes to any of these questions, and you've been feeling this way for so long that you just can't shake it and it seems normal, then you may be suffering from a mild depression known as dysthymia.

Dysthymia is a chronic form of depression that may affect as many as four million people. It usually begins in adolescence or early adulthood with at least two of the following symptoms, and lasts at least two years:

- Sad mood
- Lack of interest in activities you used to enjoy
- Weight gain or loss

- Too much sleep, or difficulty staying asleep
- Lack of energy, or restless
- Feelings of worthlessness, low self-esteem, or guilt
- Difficulty concentrating or making decisions
- Recurring thoughts of death or suicide

A recent study by the Rand Corporation indicates that even though 80 to 90 percent of people with depression who get help eventually improve, less than a third of people suffering from this illness receive proper medical treatment. The study also reveals that African Americans are especially unlikely to get treatment.

New studies from the National Institute of Mental Health show that depression increases your chances of having a heart attack. It is often highly correlated with strokes, cancer, diabetes, and premature death. Depression is also the leading cause of work disability.

And women are depressed at nearly twice the rate of men (12 percent of women versus 7 percent of men). Sadly, the leading reasons we don't get the care we need, according to the Rand study, are embarrassment about bringing up the subject and limited availability of treatment.

Because of our vulnerability to daily stresses that can trigger depression—such as encountering racism, facing economic challenges, not having a strong support network, and suffering loss of a loved one through death or divorce—it's all the more important for us to be aware of our moods. Unlike major depressive episodes and their obvious symptoms—such as difficulty getting out of bed—dysthymia is often difficult to diagnose. It robs its victims over time, but if left untreated, it can also evolve into major depression.

Today there are many successful treatments for dysthymia.

First, if you notice that you've had little energy for a while, get into therapy. You may also benefit from antidepressant medications such as Prozac, which have proven highly effective, especially when combined with therapy. (A physician or psychiatrist will have to prescribe the meds.)

You can also go the herbal route and try a supplement like Saint-John's-wort. It's best to take this or any other herbal treatments under the supervision of an herbalist or holistic physician. And always tell your doctor about any medications—including supplements—you're taking.

It's important to remember that feeling blue isn't natural, or something you have to live with. By getting help—through therapy, medication, or both—you *can* feel better.

For more information, read Julia A. Boyd's book *Can I Get a Witness? Black Women and Depression* (Plume; $11.95).

9

Daughters
of a Dream Deferred

Most often, the brightest light you can cast on chal-
lenges, dilemmas and trying times is the light within
yourself. Creating strategies to identify and chan-
nel feelings of anger, and to promote the power of your
spirit, is an invaluable part of realizing your dreams. In
this chapter, bestselling author, motivational speaker,
and certified spiritual counselor Dorothy Randall Gray
shares tips on how to redirect feelings of anger and
frustration.

I was doing OK until "the other woman" called. I was handling
this breakup. But I didn't even know there was another woman.
And she hadn't been told much about me. An almost two-year
relationship had become invisible—in just one week!

"I'm so sorry. I really didn't know," she explained. I held

the phone in one hand. In the other was a letter from my ex in which he claimed that "life was lonely" without me, and closed with the fatal "I hope we can still be friends." My angry body felt 10 degrees hotter. I wasn't feeling my spiritual side—I was thinking homicide.

I festered, called friends, and cried. I did everything but direct the anger at its source. Then I began to reason it away. I started "should-ing" on myself: "I really should not be feeling this way . . ." I began to think I wasn't entitled to my anger. Eventually I told myself I wasn't angry at all.

That happened to me a while ago, but the feelings I didn't express are still raw. Have you ever hidden your feelings on the back shelf, then wondered why they collected dust? Do you put your anger on layaway, then question why it feels as if you can never own it? Did you put it on hold so long that it hung up on you?

Anger has roots in a field of denied desires. You can't get what you want, you are not getting what you're giving, or you've lost what you had. Anger has a physical presence all its own. Have you ever walked into a room and felt angry words, even if you didn't hear them?

You don't want to seem like another "angry black woman," so you stuff these feelings where you think no one can see them. Now you're walking around with storm clouds in your soul and wondering why everyone's running for cover.

If any of this sounds like you, try these steps to help release the anger:

1. Give your anger another place to go: Write it out, or dance yourself into a sweat. Walk around the block counterclockwise stomping your feet (an African technique that asks your ancestors for help).

2. Begin to sort through the issues to determine what is important, what is the other person's, and what is yours.

3. Speak your mind when it's clear, not when it's clouded by anger.

4. Begin to change the patterns that invite anger into your life. This can be difficult and may be best done with the help of a therapist or spiritual counselor.

5. Above all, tell yourself, "I have a right to be angry." Anger denied can manifest as depression. Denial is the drug of dreams deferred.

Do you feel anger that you would like to channel? If so, what steps can you take to release that anger? Jot down your strategies and ideas in the section below. Don't forget to refer back to your notes when you need some of your own advice.

10

HOW TO LET YOUR
Inner Light Shine

*In this chapter, Dorothy Randall Gray shares tips on
how to make your inner light shine.*

"Baby, when we make love, you're going to see stars!" I proudly
proclaimed to the love of my life.

When I turned out the lights, my bedroom became a shining
wonderland of glow-in-the-dark planets and constellations.
And I was glowing like one of those fluorescent stars I'd spent
hours pasting on my ceiling.

"See?" I said, slipping under the covers.

I remember a time, though, when nothing was shining
within me or my room. Years ago, I had a roommate who kept
the utility bills in her handbag so she wouldn't forget to pay
them. Of course, she'd forget anyway, and the power was always getting turned off. The first time the lights went out, my
roommate waltzed out of the apartment declaring, "Oh well,

I've been meaning to defrost the refrigerator anyway!" and left me sitting in the dark.

When this started to become a pattern, my anger grew as much as my feelings of powerlessness. "It's her apartment," I thought to myself, "so what can I do?" As I pondered my predicament, I remembered other situations in which I had felt I had no control or had allowed someone to make me feel as if I had no right to shine. The experience also brought to mind the times I took it upon myself to hide "this little light of mine" for fear of shining too brightly. I was experiencing a personal power shortage.

So I called on spirit, asked for guidance, and realized I needed to get an apartment of my own. Meditation also helped me focus on the larger issues—taking charge of my circumstances, owning my own power, and not being afraid to use it.

Do you sometimes feel as if someone turned off your lights and you can't find the switch? Are you afraid to manifest your full potential because of what others might think? If so, you may be suffering from an inner blackout.

Here's how to turn those lights back on:

1. Ask yourself, "What's really going on here?" and "What would I do if I wasn't afraid?" Be honest with yourself; facing the truth will help you grow.

2. Use meditation or counseling, or talk to an elder or spiritual adviser, to focus on these larger issues. Then take steps to address them.

3. Affirm yourself daily by adapting the words from Nelson Mandela's inaugural address and saying them as if they were meant for you: "As I let my own light shine, I unconsciously give other people permission to do the same. My playing small does not serve the

world. There is nothing enlightened about shrinking so that other people will not feel insecure around me. I was meant to shine.I was born to make manifest the glory of God that is within me."

4. Think of yourself as a shining wonderland, then glow on with your bad celestial self!

Have you ever suffered from a personal power outage? Are you suffering from one now? If so, what steps did you—or will you—take to turn the electricity back on? Jot down your strategies and ideas in the section below.

_____

_____

_____

_____

_____

_____

_____

_____

_____

_____

_____

_____

11

Pass *the* Passion, Please!

In this chapter, Dorothy Randall Gray shares tips on how to bring passion back into your life.

I'll never forget a frustrating, unsatisfying lovemaking session I experienced years ago. After it was over, the perpetrator, who shall remain nameless, leaned back and asked smugly, "Was it good?" I confess, I wasn't as enlightened then as I am now. The shadow side of me jumped out and replied, "Was it in?"

How could someone have been so blind to *my* needs? That had happened once too often. Something inside me just gave up; it was easier not to feel anything than it was to feel hurt or frustrated. My passion plane took a nosedive.

Over the years, I've discovered that many other women take refuge behind that same wall of disillusionment. I've also learned how forceful, yet amazingly fragile, passion can be. Grief, stress, fear, worry, rejection, and depression can totally devastate the passion principle.

Passion is more than a sexual sensation. It is also defined as "boundless enthusiasm, a powerful emotion or appetite." Without access to your passion, you don't have full access to your joy. You're denied a wholeness that can make your heart sing and your soul soar. Minus passion, a voice inside you is always whispering, "There's something missing . . ."

What are you *truly* passionate about? Are you being spiritually shortchanged? If there are roadblocks on your passion path, these ideas may help to clear the way again. Begin with your outer surroundings, then slowly work your way toward your inner environment.

1. Body passion: Try wearing shoes and clothing that make you feel sensuous and not just sensible. Spray your sheets with rosewater and sleep in something soft and silky.

2. Mind passion: Take small steps toward the "I've always wanted to . . ." things that really excite you. Want to finish school? Get the catalog, take a noncredit course, talk to a counselor, visit the school, and visualize yourself as a student there. Reward yourself at every step.

3. Spirit passion: Take a passion bath. Turn off all phones and lights. Place red candles and other red items around your bathroom (red invites passion, helps you meet life's challenges, and encourages self-confidence). Put on sensuous music, run a warm bath, and scent the water with jasmine, an oil that summons love. Speak to the water: "Divine passion surrounds me, sensuous spirit enfolds me, and joy shines within

me. I am whole, I am blessed, I am . . ." Now soak for a while, lose yourself in the music, and feel the words seep into your pores. Then, at the end of a night of high-quality solitude, whisper to yourself, "The passage to my passion is clear, and I am at peace."

Is passion missing from your life? Have you developed ideas—or heard or read suggestion—on how to bring passion back into your life ? Jot down your ideas in the section below.

_____

_____

_____

_____

_____

_____

_____

_____

_____

_____

_____

_____

12

THE CONNECTION BETWEEN

Post-Traumatic Slavery Disorder

AND DEPRESSION IN

BLACK WOMEN

Clinical psychologist and NiaOnline columnist Jeffrey Gardere, Ph.D., is the author of Love Prescription: Ending the War Between Black Men and Women *and* Practical Parenting, *co-authored with Montel Williams. Here he explains why the legacy of slavery continues to wreak havoc on black women's well-being and how we can overcome its lingering and profound effects.*

Levels of depression among black women are off the charts. A 2001 study from the Black Women's Health Imperative indicates that up to 60 percent of African American women show signs of depression. And according to recent testimony given to the American Psychological Association, women who are members of ethnic-minority groups have a greater risk than white women of having their depression go unrecognized and be inadequately treated. This puts nonwhite women at even higher risk for continued depression and exposure to a host of other illnesses.

As Women's eNews correspondent Shauna Curphey reports, "In California, African American women have the shortest life expectancy among women of all racial and ethnic groups in the state. They also have the highest mortality rate [from] heart disease and stroke and the highest prevalence of high blood pressure and obesity." She goes on to indicate that mental-health issues, especially depression, may be a key reason for these elevated statistics, not just in California but throughout the United States.

It is obvious that depression is not only a serious problem among African American women, its prevalence can also be life-threatening. Studies have documented the reason for such high rates of untreated depression: the persistent taboo within the African American community against discussing mental-health issues. Black women fear that if they talk about their depression, either no one will listen or they'll be shunned. But I believe the greater question is: Why do black women become depressed in the first place? Researchers have varying explanations for what causes depression. It is most likely a combination of genetic, biological, and environmental factors. For women in particular, additional causes are hormonal imbalances, menopause, and chronic gynecological illnesses. There has not, however, been enough research documenting the role of race as a contributor to African American women's depression—particularly as it relates to the legacy of slavery. I firmly believe that this legacy expresses itself in post-traumatic slavery disorder, or "(our)PTSD," the term that I have coined for this mental-health disorder, which I have written about extensively, especially in my book *Love Prescription: Ending the War Between Black Men and Women.*

Famed psychiatrist Alvin Poussaint, M.D., was the first clinician to identify and begin working with this concept, calling it post-traumatic slavery syndrome. But because (our)PTSD is not yet considered a clinical disorder by the mental-health and medical establishments, its effects have not been measured. It is my firm belief, however, that it is a real phenomenon and does create or contribute to the depression of black women, perhaps to a significant degree.

Post-traumatic stress disorder (PTSD), the clinically recognized and documented predecessor to post-traumatic slavery disorder, is a psychological reaction to being exposed to a traumatic event, such as a mugging, rape, car accident, or police brutality—anything that should not normally happen, even in a less-than-perfect world. Symptoms include anxiety, depression, flashbacks, and avoidance behaviors. With post-traumatic slavery disorder, the traumatic event was slavery! The black people who first experienced slavery were kidnapped, brutalized, raped, and coerced into human bondage. As a result, they exhibited symptoms of post-traumatic stress disorder, including nightmares, rage, and a complete destruction of their self-esteem. They also developed inordinate amounts of anxiety and depression.

If we fast-forward to African Americans of today, many of them the descendants of slaves, we find that they suffer the same symptoms of post-traumatic slavery disorder as their ancestors because of collective memories, commu-

How often do you think about your race?

Constantly	(36.3%)
Do not know	(20.1%)
Daily	(18.1%)
Hourly	(1.2%)
Monthly	(5.4%)
Never	(8.1%)
Weekly	(9.2%)
Yearly	(1.7%)

Data drawn from a total of 906 respondents.

Source: NiaOnline CAP

nicated history (in other words, passed-down behaviors and beliefs from one generation to another), and their exposure to the aftermath of slavery: day-to-day racism. This racism continues to fuel a prejudiced society, causing economic, social, and psychological atrophy in the black community and black consciousness.

Daily racism exposes black women, who arguably occupy the bottom rung of America's social ladder, to relentless disrespect, abuse, and a lack of opportunity in white society, resulting in an inordinate amount of stress. This stress may put them at high risk for developing (our)PTSD and its major symptom, depression. It may well be, therefore, that post-traumatic slavery disorder is partly responsible for the depression that manifests itself in the lives of black women in the following ways:

Dysfunctional Relationships

Black people were forced into slavery and treated as animals. Male slaves were beaten at will, and their females were sexually violated by the white masters. This experience not only resulted in post-traumatic slavery disorder among individuals but, in turn, severely affected the black family as a unit. The anxiety and depression from (our)PTSD has contributed to maladaptive behaviors that have been passed down through the generations, negatively affecting the way black men and women view themselves and relate to each other and resulting in significant family and relationship dysfunction. Therefore, not only do black women have to deal with their own issues of inequity in society, but they must also contend with the stress of their damaged families and mating relationships.

I firmly believe that in fulfilling the role of the maternal figure, black women also shoulder the burden of (our)PTSD–related issues in black men—especially the anger! The emasculation of the black man didn't just happen during slavery; it continues every single day in society. Black men who do not have a healthy outlet for their frustrations may act out their anger through self-destructive behaviors such as promiscuity, crime, and drug and alcohol abuse. But healthy outlets or not, most often the anger is brought home and—consciously or unconsciously—is expressed and acted out at home (perhaps one reason for the high rate of domestic violence in black homes). In a 1998 study by the Annenberg School for Communication at the University of Pennsylvania, 42.9 percent of the 405 African American respondents said that they had strong reason to believe that a woman they knew had been physically abused by her husband or boyfriend in the past year. According to the U.S. Department of Justice, approximately one in three African American women is abused by a husband or partner during her lifetime.

The black woman, therefore, isn't just the black man's sounding board; too often, she is also his emotional or physical punching bag. Take the case of Kareem and Janice:

Kareem, an engineer for a power-supply company, had been passed over for promotions several times by a white supervisor who consistently promoted white employees with less tenure and qualifications. Though normally a gentle, loving husband and father to his wife and family, Kareem was frustrated by what he perceived as continuing racism on the job. He unknowingly took out his emotions on Janice. Though he would never hurt her physically, his anger was overwhelming, and he became both withdrawn and dismissive with her and the children. Janice did everything in her power to try to be supportive, but she could not soothe his anger and was often peppered with insults from him.

Eventually the emotional barrage became too much for Janice, causing her to become frustrated and angry herself. Consequently,

Janice developed severe depression. She kept her emotional pain to herself, in part because she didn't want to betray Kareem by telling their business, but also because she felt ashamed at not being able to handle the situation within the family. Eventually she became suicidal and swallowed an overdose of pills. It was at this point that they came to my attention, with each receiving individual mental-health treatment and both enrolled in couples counseling. She is now stable, and they are both doing better individually and in their marriage, having addressed how (our)PTSD has affected their lives, and what they need to do in acknowledging and confronting it as a potent force.

The Emotional Pain of Being an African American Mom

Post-traumatic slavery disorder affected not only black men and women and their descendants but also the white master and his children. Their horrendous treatment of black people became a learned behavior, but the hatred and disdain they felt for black people also became an emotional liability. To be rooted in this kind of thinking and behavior is self-destructive, and the result in society is day-to-day racism, conscious and unconscious, as well as institutional racism. Even worse is the way that black children are perceived and treated within that environment. As mothers, black women must raise their children in a society that values the lives of black children less than it does those of white children. And too often, African American mothers must endure the stress of watching their sons and daughters not only being treated as inferior but also being brutalized.

We recently witnessed the shocking images of a five-year-old black girl who was videotaped by Florida school administrators as she was throwing a temper tantrum and later as she was handcuffed by police officers (who also shackled her legs in their police car). I spent time with this little girl and her mother, interviewing them and doing some counseling, while they were in New York City to tape the television news series *A Current Affair*. I can honestly tell you that each time the mother viewed the tape of her daughter being handcuffed, tears would well up in her eyes, and the pain of seeing her daughter emotionally and physically brutalized was written across her face. I am convinced that this woman will experience post-traumatic slavery disorder and its accompanying depression.

I also watched this tape with other African American women who began to cry at the events they witnessed. Almost all of them said that this is what it must have been like when our women and children were being assaulted by the slave master. The point is that it's stressful enough being a mother in today's society, but it's much more stressful being a black mother, constantly fighting for the equitable education and treatment of her children. That mother's stress is a certain cause of post-traumatic slavery disorder.

Black Women's Unequal Treatment in the Workplace

We frequently hear about the so-called glass ceiling that white women face on the job. Although they may be just as qualified as their white male counterparts, they are cut off from achieving parity in pay and advancement. Quite often these women have sued their companies because of the degrading and traumatic experience of being refused their rightful promotions. To add insult to injury, they are often devalued and considered more for their sexuality than for their intellectual abilities.

Well, if white women are limited by a glass ceiling, it stands to reason that black women are facing a "steel curtain" when it comes to having their skills and potential for promotion acknowledged! Black women aren't just kept from occupational advancement; they are frequently degraded, embarrassed, and traumatized by their superiors. Psychologically, because of the historical relationship between white masters and female slaves, black women

Within the past 12 months at work, do you feel you were treated worse than, the same as, or better than people of other races?	
Same as other races	(36.1%)
Worse than other races	(26.8%)
Worse than some races, better than others	(16.9%)
Do not know	(8.3%)
Unemployed or self-employed	(6.3%)
Have only encountered people of the same race	(3.3%)
Better than other races	(2.3%)
Data drawn from a total of 909 respondents.	

Source: NiaOnline CAP

may be perceived as "concubines." The sexuality and attractiveness of the black female employee can feed into the unconscious fantasies of an unenlightened boss, keeping him from recognizing her intellectual and professional competence.

If white women can be traumatized by mistreatment because of their gender, then certainly black women can develop post-traumatic slavery disorder from the double whammy of being female and black. Consider the case of Sonya:

Sonya, a young executive at an advertising company, was recently referred to me for psychological evaluation because of workplace sexual harassment. She was the brightest and best at this company. She had won several awards and was bringing in contracts from companies who were enamored with her work. Though she had been promoted as the team leader of her group, that's as far as she was to go in her company. Her talent had received much attention from her male bosses, but more attention was being paid to her very attractive appearance. It became quite clear from comments that they

Within the past 30 days, have you felt emotionally upset (for example, angry, sad, or frustrated) as a result of how you were treated based on your race?	
No	(54.4%)
Yes	(42.3%)
Not sure	(3.3%)

Data drawn from a total of 903 respondents.

Source: NiaOnline CAP

made that in order for her to advance fur-ther, she would have to become physically involved with certain superiors. Sonya, who was a fiercely proud African American woman, would not subject herself to what she viewed as the master-female slave tryst repeating itself. She made it clear that she wasn't willing to play that game. The anxiety, frustration, and anger she felt in seeing her potential being stifled ulti-mately led to severe depression. Sonya had to take extended sick leave, which put her in a position to be fired. Eventually she sought psychiatric treatment and is now involved in a lawsuit against the company.

Recovering From the Trauma

Of course there are curative steps that can be taken to help re-solve (our) PTSD and its depressive effects on women of color. Try taking these measures:

Consider for yourself whether post-traumatic slavery disorder is a real psychological disorder that may be affecting your life by causing depression and, thus, taking a toll on your day-to-day functioning. If you believe that it is, seek out counseling, and possibly medication, immediately. Break the silence. Find a good clinician or support group to whom you can verbalize your emotional pain. (The Association of Black Psychologists has a directory at abpsi.org/search_referrals.htm, but the group does not verify the credentials of anyone on the list. All psychologists must meet certain certification or licensing re-quirements, and you should always check a psychologist's cre-dentials with your state licensing board.) Your loved ones and friends will not ostracize you or think less of you. If they do, shame on them! And if you are involved in a destructive relationship, make sure not only that the two of you receive couples counseling but also that your partner gets help for his or her issues and possible post-traumatic slavery disorder. The fact is, you do not have to live with untreated depression and anxiety caused by (our) PTSD—or any other situation or syndrome.

Instead of suffering through the depression, in addition to getting professional help, redirect your energies to becoming empowered to solve the problems causing the injustice, not just for yourself and family but also for the community. Kadiatou Diallo, the mother of Amadou Diallo, fought the good fight to make the legal system address the brutal death of her beloved son who, though unarmed, was shot 41 times by New York City police officers. She has become an advocate to make sure that no other mother has to bury her son over a racial injustice. Fight for equity in your child's school as well as in your community's school system. In the workplace, document any perceived prejudice, inequity, or sexual harassment, and make sure these situations are addressed immediately, each and every time.

Analyze and discuss with loved ones exactly how post-traumatic slavery disorder affects your life and romantic relationships as a woman of color and, if relevant, as a mother and career woman. Then take steps to address these issues, not only with professional medical help but also with the support of partners and family. As a psychologist, but more importantly as a man of color, I believe it is important

> **Within the past 30 days, have you experienced any physical symptoms (for example, an upset stomach, tensing of your muscles, or a pounding headache) as a result of how you were treated based on your race?**
>
> | | |
> |---|---|
> | **No** | **(72.3%)** |
> | **Yes** | **(23.5%)** |
> | **Not Sure** | **(4.2%)** |
>
> Data drawn from a total of 904 respondents.
>
> *Source: NiaOnline CAP*

for us as black men and women to communicate with and support each other through our shared post-traumatic slavery disorder and the emotional aftermath. Let's work it out as friends and lovers, not as adversaries. In time, you'll find that the depression and any other emotional issues will get better.

13

At-Home Pampering

Everyday life can be tough on all of us. Try spending as little as 15 minutes or as long as an entire leisurely day enjoying one of these soothing and rejuvenating treatments. After all, you've earned it!

Bathing Beauty

Much more than just a way to get clean, baths increase blood flow to the muscles and skin for relaxation and a radiant glow. Once the kids have gone to bed, or maybe before they wake up, take 20 minutes to light some candles, pop in a Sade CD, and soak. Not only will the stress wash off of you, but depending on your choice of herbs and oils, the healing effects can be considerable. (One suggestion: Throw in three chamomile tea bags for a good night's rest, or a cup of Japanese sake to detoxify and refresh skin.)

Check out the salts and oils from the Red Flower line,

inspired by Japanese bathing rituals and designed to improve the body's flow of energy. Or release your inner child with one of the original bath "bombs" by Lush (our favorite is Lavender Blissard; $4 to $6).

Get Steamed

It is incredible what wonders can come from draping a towel over your head and standing over a steaming bowl of water. Herbal steams are great for releasing toxins from pores and improving circulation.

Three Tips to Avoid Burnout

Take off the Superwoman cape! Despite the fact that everyone expects you to do it all, you can't—nor should you try to! Make sure to carve out some "me" time on a regular basis. One trick of successful working moms is to wake up an hour earlier, when everyone else is still asleep, and devote that time to a morning walk, yoga, reading, or whatever brings you peace of mind and better health.

Get organized! A disorganized life creates extra stress and makes it harder to carve out time to exercise or relax. You may think you don't have the time to put your affairs in order, but once you do it will free up a lot of extra time you didn't even know you had. Get a handheld PDA to help you keep track of your schedule and tasks, or simply write out a weekly checklist with pen and paper. To make sure that everything in your environment has a place of its own, make a trip to the Container Store or any other retail outlet specializing in space organization products. Use the extra time you've created to engage in your favorite stress relief activity.

Get a good night's sleep! Getting adequate sleep not only helps you to approach the world refreshed and to handle your business more efficiently, but some experts say it also makes it easier to maintain a healthy weight by curbing your appetite. Even if you can't carve out more time to sleep, you can boost the quality of your shut-eye by minimizing the distractions in your sleeping area (new mothers, we realize this may be an impossible challenge for you). Break the habit of falling asleep with the television on, or even reading before you go to sleep. Also: eating within three hours of bedtime is a no-no. If your stomach is still at work, how do you expect the rest of you to fall asleep?

Add a handful of herbs or flowers (a cup of fresh rose petals will draw out dirt while lulling you with its intoxicating scent) or eight drops of essential oils (a rosemary-and-peppermint combination removes impurities and clears sinuses) to a bowl of boiling water and then exhale and relax for 10 minutes. Pick up several essential oils at the Body Shop ($10 to $14) so that you'll have a selection at hand.

Honey Child

Some Native American cultures traditionally use honey to cleanse the skin after a person has undergone a spiritual journey. So it seems like the ideal ingredient to add to a beauty treatment. Heat a quarter-cup of honey in the microwave (20 seconds is sufficient), then mix with a tablespoon of cornmeal. Apply to face and neck, sit back and relax for 10 minutes, and remove with a warm washcloth.

Honey is a natural humectant (meaning it attracts and retains moisture), so you'll be rewarded with both soft skin and a soothed spirit. Follow with Carol's Daughter Honey Butter ($12) for head-to-toe satisfaction.

Cosmetic Enhancements

Here are three quick tips that will leave you looking refreshed and revitalized:

1. Keep eyebrows groomed as an instant way to look polished.
2. Using your fingers, tap a rose-toned blush onto the apples of your cheeks for a fresh-faced glow.
3. Wake up your face and draw attention to your lips with a deep plum or red lipstick. (Look for shades with a yellow or gold undertone.)

14

The Challenge *of the* Thirties

ACCEPTING THE BATTLE

During her thirties, NiaOnline editor-in-chief Sheryl Huggins discovered that the battle for better health is continual—and not always encouraging. In this chapter, she shares why it is nonetheless worthwhile to wage.

Remember that television commercial for an anti-aging skincare product where a beautiful, youthful-looking woman is taking a lie-detector test? She tells a few obvious lies (for instance, answering "no" when asked, "Do you frequently date younger men?"), and naturally the needle on the lie detector jumps like crazy. Then the interviewer asks her, "How old are you?" A sly smile plays on her lips as she answers, "29." The needle draws a line as flat as an ironing board. The presumption is that she is actually over 30, but using the anti-aging product makes her look twentysomething and allows her to lie about her age convincingly.

Many black women in their thirties (and far beyond), including me, can relate to this scenario. No store-bought beauty product gets the credit, however. As they say, "Black don't crack." Smooth, wrinkle-resistant skin is our genetic legacy, allowing us to pass as younger women if we choose to. In my case, reasonably healthy eating and exercise habits adopted in my early thirties allow me to maintain the illusion at age 39 . . . on the outside. As is the case with many black women, the inside tells a different story.

My thirties introduced me to high blood pressure, gall bladder disease, a burst appendix, a benign tumor, fibroids, weight battles, and more. Sure, I had heard all the warnings aimed toward African Americans by the health care community, such as, "African Americans have the highest rate of hypertension of any ethnic group, so watch your weight and get your blood pressure checked." I even knew that certain conditions which plague our community, such as high blood pressure and diabetes, run in my family. I just never truly believed that the warnings applied to me—especially since I looked healthy and baby-faced. Even when I was carrying an extra 30 pounds, I wore it well enough to attract appreciative glances from the opposite sex. Many brothers prefer their women thick anyway, I knew.

Then during my thirty-second year came frequent headaches, which sent me to my doctor. A check of my blood pressure revealed that it was borderline high according to 1990s standards: 140/90. (The American Heart Association [AHA] now advises people to keep their blood pressure at 120/80 or below. A systolic pressure reading—the upper number—of 120-139 is considered to be "prehypertensive," as is a diastolic pressure reading—the lower number—of 80-89.) My doctor advised that I lose a little weight and that we monitor my blood pressure over the next year before considering putting me on medication to control it.

In the meantime, I tried to cut back on how much salt I ate, because too much salt intake raises blood pressure in some people. I stopped cooking with salt, or shaking it into my food during meals. However, I was still eating lots of processed foods with high sodium content, such as frozen dinners, deli meats, and canned soups. I was especially fond of olives, Chinese takeout food, and sushi drenched in "light" soy sauce. I also struggled to lose a few pounds by stepping up my exercise routine of jogging in the park, with limited success. You see, I love to eat big portions, especially late at night. I also love to run, but I hate to push myself. Meanwhile, my blood pressure climbed. At one point, I actually had a reading of 165/110—the lower reading being in the "severe" range, according to the AHA. At that point, my doctor and I decided that I should go on medication to lower it.

Which is what I did for several months, until the bottom fell through my world: my father was suddenly diagnosed with Stage 4 lung cancer, and within a few weeks of entering the hospital for what we had thought was a blood clot, he was gone. Two months later, my gall bladder unexpectedly burst, requiring emergency surgery. (Being overweight is also a risk factor for gall bladder disease, I discovered too late.) In many ways, I had hit bottom.

The stress of grieving, coupled with the post-surgery recovery process, immediately melted 10 pounds off of me. Despite the pain and trauma I'd been through, I sensed the momentum, and I tried to capitalize on it. I soon lost another 20 pounds through a more sensible diet and a stepped-up running routine. In the chaos surrounding my emergency surgery, I had forgotten to keep taking my high blood pressure pills. I never took them again—and eventually, I didn't need to.

I would like to say that my health problems ended there, or that I kept all the weight off, but that isn't the case. The next few years would see me through more weight swings, more stress, and more hospital visits, until I finally achieved equilibrium—at least for now. For the past couple of years I have maintained the same weight range—30 pounds or more below my peak—and I have avoided any hospital visits. I exercise with about the same frequency, just much harder. After years of struggling, I also figured out how to eat less and more healthily without feeling deprived. Now I read the nutrition facts labels on the back of every processed food item I buy to check the sodium, fat, and sugar content. However, I still battle to stay on course. I've resigned myself to the fact that staying healthy will never be effortless. The notion that choosing health and wellness is a lifelong effort is very real, and sometimes it can wear you down.

For instance, just when you think you're finally getting a leg up on the quest for better health, they hit you with another set of guidelines.

Take the dietary and fitness guidelines released by the federal government during the winter of 2005. Check them out at Health.gov. You thought the previous standard of getting 30 minutes a day of moderate exercise was a challenge? Now they say 30 minutes a day makes you a slacker, with a full *hour a day* required to keep off extra pounds!

"Who has time for even 30 minutes a day?" I asked a fresh-faced personal trainer at my gym one evening not long after. At the time, I was on a treadmill taking a fitness test to measure my body's aerobic efficiency—in other words, how well my heart pumps oxygen to the rest of my body when I exercise.

I'll admit, like the lady in the commercial who fooled the lie detector, I was feeling pretty sure of myself. These days I generally work out three or four times a week, and when I run, I usually log four to seven miles. My blood pressure readings are now generally 130/80 or below. I won't be walking a runway anytime soon, but I *look* reasonably fit. Given where I had been several years ago, I'd call that real progress.

"Still, with all that, I don't average 30 minutes a day of moderate exercise—much less 60 minutes," I confessed to Mr. Fresh Face, who nodded with a smile and said, "I know; that's a lot of time for the average person."

"I mean, it's tough enough for me with my job; but women with partners and children have it even tougher. How are you supposed to find the time?" I continued. "I try to work it into my daily routine; for instance, as a New Yorker, I walk a lot (taking my car into the city is too much of a hassle on most weekdays, so I ride the subway). When I have errands on the weekends, I'll include them in my running plans."

"Yes, that seems to be the key," he said. "It has to be a natural part of your day." Then he increased the incline and speed on the treadmill and asked me how I was doing.

"Fine," I answered. I could definitely feel my heart pumping and the pleasant ache of muscular effort in my legs, but it was all good. I felt I could keep on going for an hour at least.

"Your heart rate has reached the 65 percent range," he said, meaning that at about 120 beats per minute I was 35 percent away from the fastest rate at which my heart should be able to beat. The maximum rate is about 180 beats per minute for the average person my age (the AHA suggests you subtract your age from 220 in order to find your maximum). Staying in the 65 percent-to-85 percent zone would help me burn fat and maintain my weight.

After about a minute, he announced, "Eighty-five percent. OK, let's slow you down and see how long it takes you to return to your starting heart rate of about 95 beats per minute." The incline and speed were reduced, and I continued chatting with him about the challenges of convincing women to take their health more seriously—all the while keeping an eye on the pulse-rate monitor. Somehow, it got stuck around 110. Is that good? I wondered, knowing deep down inside that it probably wasn't.

"Oh well, let's just stop," he said, adding to my anxiety. Two flights downstairs, we went through the results in his office. After a few calculations, he showed me a chart with a set of ranges for test scores. "You are in the fair range for your age," he said, sounding hopeful. Then I spotted the fact that "fair" came below the "average" range. The only category rated lower was labeled "poor."

"You mean I scored below average?" I asked, both outraged and deflated.

"Oh, don't worry about charts and tests, as long as you feel good," he offered. "Maybe you can add another workout per week?" I rifled through my confusion for answers. Was I a slacker?

No, I concluded, because the average person doesn't actually *get* that minimum 30 minutes of daily exercise five times a week that the government recommends. Only 31 percent of us get at least either 30 minutes of light-to-moderate exercise five times a week or 30 minutes of vigorous exercise three times a week, according to the Centers for Disease Control and Prevention.

I left Mr. Fresh Face's office with a little less spring in my step, and punished myself with a vigorous workout. Then I wondered if the test had been correctly administered. Still, since then I have been feeling a little less sure of myself, but also challenged to find the right kind of regimen to kick my heart into better shape. Right now I am trying more interval training when I run, in which I vary my pace up and down during the course of each run. It's also a good technique for people who prefer to exercise by walking (see the next chapter for more advice on how to get the most out of a walking routine).

This isn't about fitting into a size 2 swimsuit or chasing a six-pack or anything else having to do with looking good on the outside—this is about holding on to good health for as long as I possibly can. It's about how much better I feel when I exercise than I feel when I don't. I may never score exceptionally well on an aerobic-efficiency test, but the alternative—life in the out-of-shape, gasping-for-air, "poor" range (been there)—doesn't appeal to me at all.

That doesn't mean that it's never tempting to throw in the towel, however. The other day, I related my story to a friend who is decidedly antiexercise. "Wow," he said. "Don't you feel discouraged? Makes you want to eat a pork chop, doesn't it? I think I have one in the fridge..."

I didn't choose the pork chop that day. Yet every day, I face a new set of choices. Do I choose a fly, polished, permed hairstyle that will fall at the first sign of moisture, or do I stick with the sweat-proof natural twists that allow me to keep up my exercise routine? Do I have that second cup of strong black coffee, or do I ask for the decaf that I know will help me sleep better at night? During my thirties, enjoying health and wellness became one such choice—a quest, really—rather than the blessing I took for granted in my twenties. I leave my thirties knowing the price to be paid for making the wrong choices.

I truly hope that *Choosing Health and Wellness* will help more African American women to make the right choice—for themselves, and the loved ones who depend on them being around another day. Please do not be fooled by how well we look on the outside. Do not let the ample warnings about the threats to our health go in one ear and out the other. This is the time—especially for those of us in our thirties and beyond—to work on what's inside: physically, mentally, and spiritually.

PART 4

LOVING AND HONORING

THE WOMAN IN YOU

15

WHAT YOU SHOULD KNOW
About Pap Tests

Keeping healthy is a habit you learn. One of the key components of staying healthy is to understand the importance of Pap tests: what are they and how does regular testing benefit you? This chapter shares important tips on what you should know about Pap tests.

It's critically important that each of us have an annual Pap test. Though the vast majority of the 50 million women who have the test each year receive normal results, another 2 million do not.

Pap smears are tests designed to detect precancerous cells that can lead to cervical cancer, one of the most preventable diseases. Sadly, though, more than half of women who develop cervical cancer delayed getting a Pap test for three years or more. And the stats for black women are especially sobering:

According to the American Cancer Society, our death rate from cervical cancer is more than twice the national average.

It's best to be well informed about the test when you go for your gynecological exam. Here are some frequently asked questions about the Pap test.

What Is a Pap Smear?

Formally known as the Papanicolaou test, Pap smears are cell samples gathered during a pelvic exam that detect the presence of cancer or precancerous cells in the cervix.

During your exam, your doctor will insert a speculum (you know, that instrument that looks like a plastic curling iron) into your vagina to open the canal slightly. This makes for easier access to the cervix. The physician then inserts a long, cotton-tipped applicator and rubs it against the cervix. The applicator is used to spread the sample onto a slide, which is sent to a lab for testing.

During the exam, some women feel slight discomfort or pressure. But remember: It's brief. You may also experience slight spotting after the exam.

How Often Should I Get a Pap Smear?

For most women, once a year is fine. But if you have a history of abnormal Pap results, are taking birth control pills, or have recurring urinary-tract infections, you may have to have the test more often. If you put off your exam, you greatly raise your risk of going undetected not only for cervical cancer but also for some sexually transmitted diseases.

When Is the Best Time to Get a Pap Test?

If you have menstrual periods, the best time for a Pap exam is during the two weeks following the end of your flow. If you've reached menopause, you can schedule your Pap test anytime. It's also best to abstain from sexual activity and avoid using vaginal douches or lubricants for 48 hours before the exam.

What Happens If a Test Comes Back With Abnormal Results?

Don't panic! Abnormal results do not automatically mean that you have cancer. In fact, there are varying degrees of results:

Class I: Benign or normal. This is a test that comes back with no abnormal cells. You'll need to come back in a year to repeat the test.

Class II: Benign reactive. Abnormal but benign cells were found. No malignant (cancerous or precancerous) cells were found. Best to repeat the Pap test in three to six months.

Class III: Atypical squamous cells. Abnormal or atypical cells are found, but they aren't necessarily cancerous. You'll need another Pap test in three to six months. If the results are abnormal again, your health-care provider may want to biopsy some tissue.

Class IV: Dysplasia. Samples indicate there are precancerous cells but not necessarily a malignancy. Your physician will probably order a biopsy and ask you to repeat the Pap smear test in three to six months.

Class V: Malignant. A biopsy confirms that the cells are cancerous and malignant. Your physician will discuss all options with you, including surgery to remove the cancerous cells.

How Accurate Are Pap Smears?

Pap smears are very accurate at catching any early abnormalities. In a study conducted by the National Cancer Institute, Pap tests identified up to 96.3 percent of women who had precancerous or cancerous cells and needed treatment. The study also indicates that the test can eliminate the 99.5 percent of women who don't need treatment.

How Much Do Pap Smears Cost?

They aren't expensive—typically around $50—and are often covered by insurance.

For more information about Pap tests, visit the National Cancer Institute website page on Pap tests at http://cis.nci. nih.gov/fact/5_16.htm.

16

ARE YOU AT RISK

for the **Human Papillomavirus?**
(HPV)

At some point, more than 80 percent of sexually active women will contract genital human papillomavirus (HPV), America's most common sexually transmitted disease (STD). There are more than 30 forms of genital HPV, according to the Centers for Disease Control and Prevention (CDC).

Many strains don't cause any health problems or symptoms, although two cause genital warts. Several can lead to cervical cancer, which, while scary and the second-most-common cancer among women, can almost always be detected with regular Pap smears. HPV can also cause rare cancers of the vulva, vagina, anus, and penis.

There is no medical cure for any form of HPV. Even when genital warts are removed, doctors can't eliminate the virus that caused them. Fortunately, the immune system usually eradicates the disease, a process that may take several months or even years, during which time the person is contagious and probably doesn't know it.

Want to protect yourself from the consequences of genital HPV? Follow the tips we outline here.

When you have sex, make it safer. Minimize your number of sexual partners. Even if you use condoms religiously, realize that you're not completely safe; the virus can be transmitted anywhere within the area that panties or boxer shorts would cover. However, condoms do reduce your risk of cervical cancer, according to Planned Parenthood.

Be on the lookout for genital warts. Genital warts are contagious, so do try to avoid them; however, the HPV strain that causes them doesn't cause cancer or other types of warts. Ask your partners if they have ever had sex with someone who has had either genital warts or HPV—or if they've ever experienced either condition personally. Of course, they won't know for certain, but asking can help reduce your chances of exposure.

Do not have sex if you observe on yourself or your partner grayish, flesh-colored, or darker-colored bumps on or around the anus, penis, scrotum, groin, or thigh (they may also appear inside the vagina or anus or on the cervix, in which case you won't see them). The bumps may be raised, flat, or cauliflower-shaped, small or large, alone or in clusters.

Eat foods rich in beta-carotene and folic acid. Because there is no medical cure for HPV, keep your immune system strong. Planned Parenthood says the immune system can wipe out most forms in six months. It recommends eating plenty of yellow and orange fruits and vegetables such as mangoes, carrots, corn, and squash, which contain cancer-fighting beta-carotene, and dark-green leafy vegetables like spinach, which are rich in immune-strengthening folic acid.

Take care of yourself by getting a Pap smear. Have one annually if you are sexually active; however, in no case should you wait longer than three years between tests (ask your provider how often you need one). Although Pap smears cannot detect HPV itself, they alert your OB-GYN to the presence of abnormal cervical cells. She or he can then treat the cells so they don't turn cancerous.

If you're 30 or older and want to play it safe, request an HPV test, which, performed along with a Pap smear, increases the likelihood that cervical cancer will be caught early. If you don't have health insurance or cannot afford a Pap smear, call your local health department to learn where low-cost health care is available near you.

Follow up if your Pap results are abnormal. If your doctor tells you the Pap smear found abnormal cell changes (sometimes called dysplasia, precancerous cells, or cervical warts), don't panic or bury your head in the sand. According to the National Cancer Institute, only a small percentage of women who get HPV actually develop cervical cancer; the immune system usually kills the virus.

To make sure your cervix stays healthy, your doctor may order repeat or additional tests, treat the cervix with an antibiotic cream, or order a colposcopy (a procedure that allows the physician to view the cervix through a microscope) or, rarely, a biopsy (removal of a tissue sample).

Stop smoking. Smoking increases the risk of cervical cancer among women who have had HPV—as if you needed another reason to quit.

Reduce Your Risk
of Cancer

According to the American Cancer Society, half of cancer deaths are preventable. In this chapter, Philadelphia-based writer Hilary Beard describes the steps she took to lower her risk of developing cancer and details steps you can take to reduce your chances of developing breast and colon cancers—two of the top five cancers that affect black women—as well as lung, uterine, and pancreatic cancers.

Mommy caught her breast cancer early. When she first felt an unusual burning sensation in her breasts, the malignancy was too small to be detected by a mammogram. Her doctors insisted it was all in her head. Fortunately, she knew it wasn't. She insisted that something was wrong and her doctors needed to identify it. Because of her persistence, her condition was detected while there was still time to treat her and save her life.

My mother survived, but cancer is relatively common on her side of the family. Her sisters have battled ovarian, bladder, and pancreatic cancer. Her experience followed my father's devastating stroke, which left him half paralyzed and unable to work. I worried that poor health—and cancer, in particular—would be my destiny. Until, that is, I learned that I could take charge of my health and improve my fate.

Eating right, being active, and maintaining a healthy weight are important ways to reduce our risk of cancer, according to the American Cancer Society (ACS). Because of changes I've made, I know that my heart is healthy and my blood pressure and blood sugar are low. Although I don't know for sure, I am also at peace in the belief that I am avoiding the health problems that have plagued my mother and extended family.

Following are the steps I took to lower my own risk of developing cancer and suggestions on how you can take steps to reduce your chances of developing breast and colon cancers.

I started by eliminating pork, which was easy except during cookouts and trips home, when the tantalizing aroma of bacon tempted me. I didn't realize at the time that people who eat a lot of pork and red meat are at higher risk for colon cancer, but I did know that bacon, my favorite so-called white meat, is high in sodium and fat.

Instead of bacon double cheeseburgers a few times a week, I switched to Quarter Pounders with cheese. A few years later, when I learned that red meat is often high in fat, and eating a lot of it might increase my cancer risk, I grudgingly gave up burgers and switched to chicken sandwiches.

The benefits extended beyond a reduced cancer risk. The acne that had always flared up at the same time during my menstrual cycle cleared up. I also added more fruits and vegetables to my diet, which have been shown to lower the risk of several cancers, including those of the lung, mouth, esophagus, stomach, and colon. Additional benefits were seeing my previously dry skin brighten and my dandruff disappear. People commented that I looked younger.

Today I eat lots of fruit, yogurt, and whole-grain cereal for breakfast; a large green salad with plenty of colorful vegetables—topped with tuna, salmon, or organic chicken—for lunch, along with a slice of whole-grain bread with olive oil; and fish or organic chicken for dinner, often accompanied by brown rice and several types of steamed vegetables. Instead of connecting with friends at happy hour, I go walking or attend yoga class with them. My lifestyle centers around my health.

The ACS estimates that half of cancer deaths could be prevented through lifestyle changes similar to the ones I've made. The black community has started to show signs of progress: Each year since 1993, our cancer rates have been dropping at a greater rate than those of whites.

Still, we're more likely than *any* other ethnic group in the United States to die from cancer. Our lifestyles (we're more likely to be overweight and less likely to be active than the general population) could be a factor, according to the ACS, as well as our greater chances of being diagnosed later than whites (look at how hard my mother had to struggle for doctors to detect her breast cancer).

Here are specific recommendations for preventing two of the most common cancers among black women: breast and colon cancers.

Breast Cancer

Lifestyle changes: Exercising, avoiding alcohol, keeping your weight down, breast-feeding, giving birth to several children, and avoiding secondhand smoke may reduce your risk.

Get screening exams:
- Monthly breast self-exam.
- Yearly clinical breast exam.
- Annual mammogram starting at age 40.

Sister-specific advice: Although black women get breast cancer less often than white women, we are more likely to develop an aggressive form at a younger age. Some experts believe that as a precaution, black women with a family history of breast cancer should start to get annual mammograms 5 to 10 years before the age at which their relatives were diagnosed with breast cancer.

If you can't afford screening exams, call the National Breast and Cervical Cancer Early Detection Program at 888-842-6355 (select option 7). Low-cost and free screenings and treatment are available nationwide. If your sister had breast cancer, why not take part in the Sister Study (877-4-SISTER), which will be researching factors in our daily surroundings that might cause the disease? Another research project, the Southern Community Cohort Study, conducted by Vanderbilt University, the International Epidermiology Institute, and Meharry Medical College, is expected to be one of the largest health studies of black Americans ever.

Colon and Rectal (Colorectal) Cancer

Lifestyle changes: Lose excess weight; stop smoking; eat plenty of fruits, vegetables, and whole-grain foods; eat fewer high-fat foods; and get at least 3o minutes of physical activity a day, five days a week. Also, take a daily multivitamin containing folate, or folic acid, and get plenty of calcium.

Screening exam: Colonoscopy every 1o years beginning at age 45.

Sister-specific advice: The American College of Gastroenterology recommends that black folks get their first colonoscopy at 45, which is five years earlier than the age recommended for other ethnic groups. Try to avoid the flexible-sigmoidoscopy exam, which examines only the lower third of the colon. African Americans tend to develop colon cancer in the top third.

Lung Cancer

Lifestyle changes: About 9o percent of cancer deaths are caused by smoking. Kicking the habit—or avoiding smokers, if you don't smoke—is the best way to reduce your risk. Reducing the number of cigarettes you smoke each day may also help. Check the American Cancer Society website at www.cancer.org for information on smoking cessation resources.

Screening exams: Lung cancer spreads beyond the lungs before causing any symptoms. As a result, none of the screening tests—chest x-ray, computed tomography (CT) or sputum cytologic exams—has been shown to help people with lung cancer live longer. They also generate high rates of false-positive results. Talk to your doctor about the pros and cons.

Sister-specific advice: Many African Americans decline potentially lifesaving lung surgery because they mistakenly believe the myth that exposing a tumor to air spreads cancer. There is no relationship between the spread of a tumor and its exposure to air.

Cervical Cancer

Lifestyle: Quitting smoking, eating more fruits and vegetables, and limiting the number of sex partners you have (having more sex partners increases your risk of being exposed to the human papilloma virus, HPV, the family of viruses that can cause cervical cancer) and the amount of unprotected sex (although condoms don't necessarily prevent it) can all reduce your risk.

Screening: The Pap test is one of the most effective cancer screening exams. If you're over 30 you may also want to receive an HPV DNA test.

Sister-specific advice: If you've had a hysterectomy in which both the uterus and cervix have been removed, you no longer need a Pap test since you do not have a cervix—unless your hysterectomy was to treat pre-cancer or cancer; however, you should still get a pelvic exam, which examines other organs. Ask your doctor how often.

Uterine Cancer

Lifestyle: Although nobody knows the reasons why uterine cancer develops, reducing the amount of excess weight you carry and taking steps to prevent or control diabetes reduce one's risk.

Screening: Obtaining regular pelvic and rectal exams are important for detecting uterine cancer early.

Pancreatic cancer

Lifestyle: Reduce your risk by quitting smoking (believed to cause 30 percent of cases), reducing the amount of meat in your diet, especially processed meats like lunch meats and bacon, and eating a diet high in fruits, vegetables, and whole grains.

Screening: There is no screening test to prevent pancreatic cancer.

Health Insurance

Delays in diagnosis or treatment often cause people to have unnecessarily severe experiences with conditions of all types. People who don't have health insurance, in particular, may miss out on screening exams. If you don't have health insurance or are concerned about losing your existing insurance, follow these tips:

1. Visit the www.healthinsuranceinfo.net website for a free health-insurance consumer guide. The site details resources—including low-cost health insurance—available in your state, as well as your rights regarding such tricky topics as pre-existing conditions and COBRA.

2. If you are leaving your job, see if you qualify for COBRA. COBRA will allow you to stay in your group health plan for a limited time, or to get your state's continuing insurance coverage.

3. Many organizations and associations offer health insurance coverage for individuals or people who are self-employed.

4. Some insurance companies offer policies to individuals. If cost is a concern consider selecting a plan with fewer features that may be more affordable than a big employer's plan but will allow you to have some coverage.

5. Your local department of public health offers low-cost or free healthcare in an area near you.

For more detailed information on breast cancer, visit the American Cancer Society website at http://www.cancer.org and type "breast cancer" in the search field.

18

One Sister's Health Challenge

Health challenges are a reality of life, and if you haven't faced a challenge chances are you know some-one who has. This chapter describes the story of Hattie Anderson, a courageous woman who faced a critical health challenge and created an innovative founda-tion whose goal is to help women overcome similar challenges.

Hattie Anderson, the mother of an 11-year-old girl and two teenage boys, was diagnosed with inflammatory breast cancer—one of the most lethal forms of the disease—9 years ago at age 37. "I had to make some hard decisions. Do I give my life over to this disease, or do I live my life with cancer rather than worry about dying from cancer?" says Hattie.

She has done more than just choose to live life to the fullest; she has also helped other women fight back. It was during her first round of chemotherapy that she started to give monthly workshops on breast-cancer awareness and prevention. These seminars later developed into the Hattie Anderson Breast Cancer Foundation in Cerritos, California.

More than 2,000 women have gone through programs sponsored by the foundation, which has some 43 volunteers helping to provide programs on breast-cancer awareness, prevention, and early detection, as well as support groups for both the patient and her family.

These workshops are supported by the American Cancer Society, the Martin Luther King Medical Center, the Charles Drew School of Medicine, and local physicians. Taking it to the next level, Hattie now wants to buy a six-bedroom house that can be used for additional space.

Since his wife of 26 years was diagnosed with breast cancer, Donnie Anderson has become a marketing guru for breast-cancer awareness. Together the Andersons are trying to make an impact on African American women, who are dying from breast cancer at the highest rate. "And they are dying prematurely," says Donnie. "We have to break through this apathy among African American women—especially those who are under age 40—who don't want to know anything about breast cancer, so they won't do self-exams or get a mammogram."

"Most women see getting cancer as a death sentence," says Hattie. "But there is quality of life after being diagnosed with breast cancer." Hattie acknowledges that before she was diagnosed with breast cancer, it had been 11 years since she had been to an OB-GYN. She had also planned to wait until she turned 40 to get her first mammogram. Hattie has spent much of her time since the diagnosis in chemotherapy; she has had only one year and four months of remission. Here she speaks about her experience in her own words:

"I remember praying and telling God that this was too much pain to go through for nothing. Can we take this situation and turn it around for something good and let it bless someone else?

"I decided to do a one-page seminar at an inner-city library in 1993. I had two sessions with about 15 women attending. At the end of it, the ladies were asking, 'So when is your next session?' I said, 'There isn't one.' Then I thought, 'Maybe I don't have to stop doing this.'

"I continued to do one workshop a month. During the fall of 2000, around National Breast Cancer Awareness month [in October], is when I decided to do something more and expand it to a charitable foundation that offered programs.

"What I have found to be frustrating is that the women I need to reach are the ones that I have the most difficulty getting to listen. If you have a party, you can get women to come out, but they won't show up for something educational, or pertaining to their health. They don't seem to be very interested. I told them point blank: A lot of you would rather go to the mall than come here.

"Cancer has gotten a bad rap. Yes, it is a [potentially] fatal disease. But fear is the thing that is killing people. Fear is keeping women from dealing with the subject matter because they are afraid of what they might find. The notion of 'I don't want to know' exists because women think that they are going to die anyway, so why go through the pain of chemotherapy? But the hope is that chemo is just a temporary inconvenience.

"Through my past nine years of living with this disease, I have seen a lot of women in their twenties diagnosed with breast cancer. Every 13 minutes, a woman is dying of this disease. We have to care about that, and we have to do something about it. Because at least half of those deaths could have been prevented through early detection.

"There are 2.6 million women right now with breast cancer, and half of them are walking around and don't even know they have it. That means there are 1.3 million women out there that I need to find."

19

Don't Douche It!

According to the National Women's Health Information Center (800-994-9662), 37 percent of American women between the ages of 15 and 44 douche regularly, and almost half of this group do so every week. Black women are more likely than other women to douche: Sixty-six percent of us do so, according to the National Black Nurses Association (NBNA).

But although douching is a common practice, both the NBNA and the American College of Obstetricians and Gynecologists (ACOG) recommend against it. ACOG's position on douching is simple: "Do not douche," ACOG spokesperson Greg Phillips says. "It's better to let the vagina cleanse itself."

If, like many women, you douche to reduce vaginal odor or irritation or to cleanse your vagina after you've had sex or after your period, you may actually be causing the very things you are trying to prevent: You may make your hygiene worse or increase your chances of developing vaginal infections, contracting an STD—including HIV—or becoming infertile.

The vagina is "a self-cleansing organ," writes gynecologist Hilda Hutcherson, M.D., in her book *What Your Mother Never Told You About S-e-x* (Perigee; $14.95). Vaginal secretions are part of the body's natural process of keeping the vagina clean and healthy, even after you menstruate or have sex.

Each woman's vagina has a unique aroma. "The natural odor of the vagina can best be described as a pleasant musky scent," Dr. Hutcherson writes. If your discharge smells foul, is not either clear or white, or itches or burns, see a doctor, she suggests.

Douching—flushing out the vagina with water alone or a combination of water and other cleansing agents, often vinegar—is an age-old practice. Although it is commonly used to promote cleanliness, it has also been used as a birth control method and to stimulate miscarriages (for abortion).

In the United States in the 1920s and 1930s, Lysol disinfectant—yes, girl, Lysol!—was marketed to married women to help them destroy feminine "germs" and "odors." Both Lysol and Coca-Cola were squirted up the vagina because they were believed to kill sperm. Today no woman in her right mind would put Lysol in her vagina. Instead, thousands of women douche with Massengill, Summer's Eve, or solutions or treatments they mix at home.

Yet most women don't realize that douching not only can damage their reproductive health by disrupting the

---

Checklist: 5 Questions to Ask Your Gynecologist

Take this list of questions with you the next time you go to the gynecologist:

1. **How can I make sex more enjoyable?**

2. **Am I using the best contraception for me?**

3. **How can I protect myself from sexually transmitted diseases?**

4. **How can I protect my fertility?**

5. **What lifestyle choices can I make to reduce my risk of breast cancer or uterine cancer?**

elaborate "climate control" system that keeps vaginal bacteria in balance; it can also cause the very discharges, odors, and infections that women may be trying to prevent or eliminate. It can even propel bacteria and sperm into the uterus and fallopian tubes. (Note: Some women douche at the recommendation of their doctor after vaginal surgery, an episiotomy, or other reproductive medical treatment. These women should not discontinue that practice without their doctor's knowledge.)

A study published in the October 2002 issue of the journal *Obstetrics & Gynecology* found that women who douched increased their risk of developing bacterial vaginosis (BV; it's also known as nonspecific vaginitis). Those who douched once a month increased their risk by 140 percent; women who douched once a week had a risk that was more than 200 percent higher.

Bacterial vaginosis is the most common vaginal infection among women. It creates a thin, gray or even green discharge; a foul and, some women say, fishy-smelling odor; and, in some women, burning of the vulva upon urination.

BV also increases a woman's risk of pelvic inflammatory disease (PID), an infection of the uterus, fallopian tubes, and other reproductive organs. Left untreated, PID can cause chronic pelvic pain or infertility. It can even increase the likelihood of an ectopic (tubal) pregnancy, in which a fetus implants itself in the fallopian tubes instead of the uterus.

Ectopic pregnancies are more common among black women than among the general population—many experts suspect that douching is the reason for our higher rates. Because it disrupts fragile vaginal flora (beneficial microorganisms), douching also makes a woman more vulnerable to chlamydia, gonorrhea, and even HIV!

Some women douche as a form of contraception or emergency contraception. It doesn't work. According to *Our Bodies,*

Ourselves for the New Century (Touchstone; $24), douching is the least effective birth control method and actually pushes some sperm into your uterus.

If you have had unprotected sex and fear becoming pregnant, don't douche; call your gynecologist or Planned Parenthood (800-230-PLAN) immediately so you can obtain emergency contraception.

If you are worried that your discharge or odor isn't normal, share your concerns with a health care professional. She or he will help you make sure that your vagina is healthy. Then relax and allow the miraculous body you've been given to take care of itself.

20

REAL LOVE WITH DR. JEFF:

"How Do I Get Him *to* Wear a Condom?"

Clinical psychologist Jeffrey Gardere, Ph.D., is execu-
tive director of Rainbow Psychological Services in New
York City. He is also the author of Love Prescription
and former host of radio's "Conversations With Dr.
Jeff" (WWRL, 1600 AM). In this chapter, Dr. Jeff an-
swers one of the most important questions in the world
of life and love, and gives his expert advice one how to
get a brother to wear a condom.

Q: *Why is it so hard to get a brother to wear a condom, even in this*
day of AIDS and rampant sexually transmitted diseases? Every
time I get into a relationship, we start off practicing safe sex, but
sooner or later the man tries to convince me to "go bareback."

"I can't feel anything with a condom," he'll complain, or
"They're too tight on me," or he'll promise, "Just this once; I'll pull

out in time." Guys who preach safety in public will try to get around it in private. And the older the man is, the worse he fights using a condom, it seems. I once had an older boyfriend who is a professional brother tell me, "I know that all the partners I've had have been clean. People like us aren't the ones with the problem."

I know this kind of talk is ridiculous, but safe sex has nevertheless been a source of conflict in most of my relationships. Please don't tell me to drop a man just because he gives me a hard time—I'd have to become a nun, because they all do. What can I do to make it easier to keep a man (and me) satisfied, yet stand my ground?

—Seeking Safety *and* Satisfaction

Dr. Jeff: I want to congratulate you for having the courage and integrity to stand your ground thus far. I know that resisting the temptation to give in to these beggin' brothers may be hard—especially when they get hard—but stand your ground, sis. This is about your life and health.

The bottom line is that these brothers are trying to give you the ole okeydoke in order to fulfill their own selfish needs. Don't fall for their tired lyrics. When in the sex zone, some brothers will say anything to get over without using a condom.

Both you and I know that the arguments these men have been giving you are bogus:

- *"Condoms are too tight on me."* Oh, c'mon—companies make condoms in all sizes, to fit any man. Unless your guy is the size of King Kong, there's a sheath to cover his member. If they don't make a condom big enough, then you need to consider whether you want to mess with someone that huge in the first place!

- *"I can't feel anything with a condom."* Bull dinky! Latex condoms (which are the only ones you should use, by the way) come in all sorts of textures. Unless his penis is made out of leather, there should be no reason that he is not experiencing sensation. Until they make a condom that feels as good as wearing nothing at all, he will have to do with a little less sensation. Condoms are a hassle, but it's all about protection. The reality is that it's either the condom or no sex at all. Let's further put this in perspective: Ten percent of something is better than nothing at all! Besides, intercourse should not be only about the singular genital sensations; it should also be about whole-body sensations: sights, sounds, and even smell!

- *"I'll pull out in time"*—the great American lie! Sometimes our bodies just will not let us control the spirit of the boogie. And, of course, there's the danger that the man will leak pre-ejaculatory fluid, which can be just as potent as the full-bodied semen. If I were you, I wouldn't risk that chance for anything!

As far as those old male dogs are concerned, the arguments about being more mature, or a professional who is not in the risk group for having an STD, are ridiculous. Statistics have shown that the transmission of HIV does not discriminate according to educational or professional status. To cement this argument, I have two words for you: Magic Johnson! So here's my shrink-think advice:

- Inform your partners that the use of condoms is not just about your protection and health; it's also about theirs. After all, how can they be absolutely sure about your medical status or history unless they are your gynecologist? (And no, do *not* date your gynecologist!)

- Set boundaries and stick to them. Let these guys know, way before intimacy, that you have very strict rules that must and will be followed if they want to date you. And one of the most important is: Either safer sex or no sex.
- Do not put yourself in the position of negotiating condom use right before intercourse, when both of you are naked and in the heat of passion. We all know that when it comes to the sexual moment of truth, reason and good sense go out the window, along with the boxers and panties. Negotiate and talk about condom use while your clothes are on. Clothes are the best condoms around!
- Keep an assortment of condoms in your night table just in case he doesn't bring any or claims not to have one. Having your own condoms will also prevent him from using that crusty condom that has been sitting in his wallet, which may be expired and ineffective.
- Instead of being a drag or necessary evil during your encounters, make condom use a fun part of sex play. Put it on for him, using your hands or mouth or even your feet! The best part about this is that *you* have the power, not him.

Finally, sis, the deal is this: If a brother is not interested in respecting your request that he wear a condom, if he is not as compulsive and enthusiastic about it as you are, then kick him to the curb. Not only is he not respecting you and himself, but chances are he is also indulging in unsafe sex with others. Stand your ground, because the life you save may be your own.

21

REAL LOVE WITH DR. JEFF:

"I Have Herpes. Will I Find Love?"

In this chapter, Dr. Jeff answers a question about living with herpes and shares expert insights and tips.

Q: *I was in a long-term relationship during which I was monogamous. My ex, however, cheated on me, and through his infidelity I received the gift of herpes. After years of denial, shame, and the fear of being alone, I left this man.*

Now I'm back in the dating game. I recently opened up to someone I thought understood me, only to be rejected because, in his words, I was "not worth the risk" of infection. Having herpes has changed my world, and the emotional baggage is so heavy. I am seriously wondering if I will spend the rest of my life alone. What can I do to find a partner who will accept my condition?

—Damaged Goods

Dr. Jeff: First and foremost, you must get into your head that you are not "damaged goods"! You are a woman who unfortunately has become infected with the herpes virus. You must define the place of this disease in your life; you must not allow it to define who you are.

Second, and I hope that this is of some consolation to you, you are not alone. Genital herpes (HSV-2) is one of the most common sexually transmitted diseases (STDs). An estimated 45 million Americans have it—one in five people over the age of 12. Approximately 45 percent of black women are infected (the rate is about 40 percent among black men), according to the Centers for Disease Control and Prevention (CDC). So as you can see, many people are in the same boat as you and are struggling with how herpes will affect their lives and their relationships.

You are experiencing a typical emotional reaction to finding out that you have contracted genital herpes. Dealing with this situation can be devastating, especially after you've been rejected by a lover because of it. I'm sure it must have been difficult for you to reveal such an intimate and even embarrassing part of your life to your lover and then to be rejected so coldly. Shame on him!

I used to conduct support groups for young professional adults in their twenties who were in the dating mode and had just contracted genital herpes. Each and every one of the group's members experienced the same depression, anger, anxiety, and shame that you're feeling. Some were also rejected by their potential partners—which was a double emotional insult—but others were supported by their old and new loves.

Like you, initially, all of these group members defined themselves, not as people, but as people with herpes: modern lepers, damaged goods, who were doomed to carry this physical and emotional burden for the rest of their lives.

This is because herpes represents many things. First, it is a sexually transmitted disease, and despite the sexualization of America, at heart this country remains a puritanical society that views STDs as a punishment for having sex, especially outside of marriage. In addition, this STD mostly manifests itself on the genitals, which are the primary representatives and source of our sexuality and reproduction. Because we are sexual beings, when this area is involved, our self-esteem, our self-identity, and, thus, our romantic and sexual relationships can certainly be affected.

To add insult to injury, because you were infected with herpes by the unfaithfulness of your previous partner, I would venture to say that unconsciously you associate herpes with being a victim of someone's "dirty" behavior, in turn making you dirty.

Believe it or not, the group members also confronted, and dealt with, all of these issues. By the sixth week of the group, not one member felt the need to return for psychological treatment. All of them had made a personal commitment to stop being victims and instead became empowered to manage their herpes, move on with their lives, and pursue loving relationships.

This is what I had them do—and what you can do—in order to get back to the business of living their lives and pursuing romance:

• *Learn as much as you can about herpes.* Knowledge is power, and it helps reduce the fear of the unknown. Also hook up with a gynecologist who not only will discuss treatment options but also will be a good ear for your questions and concerns.

- *Find a support group.* The National Herpes Resource Center has information about support groups across North America. You can also seek support from a friend who has dealt with having herpes and talk, talk, talk! Not only will the communication be healthy and freeing, but you will also learn how another person dealt with having herpes, which will give you tried-and-true strategies for getting through this trauma. Talking to others who have been infected lets you know that you are not alone.

- *Stop letting herpes define who you are.* You are not a herpes-infected individual; you are a woman who happens to have herpes. It is not your whole life, just one small aspect of it. Write this down, say it to yourself every day, and make it an affirmation—even pray for the strength to accept this fact. In time you will find that the "herpes baggage" has become much lighter, and you will stop searching for individuals to accept you as "damaged goods" or a charity case, because you are neither of these things.

- *Don't mention herpes right away.* Although it is important to tell any potential lover about your situation, don't reveal it unless you're sure that things are heading toward sex, intimacy, or a real relationship. When you've met the person with whom you want to become intimate, let him know about your condition after you discuss your respective health histories. Just in case he doesn't know that much about herpes, come with information and brochures in hand. One of the support group members I counseled would take her potential lovers to her doctor to get educated about herpes; you can do the same.

All that being said, you will still run into guys who may not think you are worth the risk of their getting herpes. Think about it, though: These are probably the same guys who would abandon you if you were raped or in any other situation that required their understanding, help, and love. Your having herpes can be a sort of litmus test as to whether a guy you want to get involved with is really worth it! Anyone who is mature enough to deal with your having herpes may be there for you when the chips are down.

Finally, I know that you are devastated right now, but trust me, even without following my advice, eventually you would deal with this situation in a healthier way. You are still in emotional shock, but like every crisis in one's life, this too shall pass. You will not end up alone. Never forget that you are valuable, smart, and beautiful, and like every person I have counseled about herpes or any other STD, you will make it through. I promise!

PART 5

STAYING FIT AND FABULOUS

22

WHAT'S THE BIGGEST THREAT
to Black Women's Health?

Sheryl Huggins is the editor-in-chief responsible for running the day-to-day operations of the black women's online community NiaOnline.com. She is also vice president of information services for NiaOnline's parent company, Nia Enterprises, and co-editor of The Nia Guide *series of books. Huggins' career in media and communications spans more than 15 years, during which she has been a magazine publisher and entrepreneur, a newspaper reporter, a magazine editor, a business news writer, a marketing communications executive, and more. She received her B.A. degree in history from the University of Pennsylvania and an M.S. degree in journalism from Columbia University. A Brooklyn, New York resident for more than 14 years, she attempts to stay in shape and relieve stress by running in local parks. In this chapter, she shares her research and insights on the biggest challenges and threats to black women's health.*

Fifty-percent of African American women over age 20 are obese, compared to one-third of all American women.
Source: National Center of Health Statistics, 2002

"The next time you pick up a fork, use it for self-defense, and not self-destruction."
 Patricia Davidson, M.D., FACP
 Cardiologist, Washington Medical Center

In the spring of 2003 I attended a historic conference on black women's health that was held on Capitol Hill in Washington, DC. Led by the Black Women's Health Imperative (BWHI), a few hundred legislators, academics, health care professionals, community activists, insurance company executives and other concerned parties convened on the fitting date of April 11 (4-11) at the newly opened Barbara Jordan Conference Center to discuss the state of health and health care for African American women. NiaOnline was among the partner organizations participating in this kick-off to a national dialogue on how to improve black women's health.

If we took nothing else away from the National Colloquium on Black Women's Health, we took this away: The number-one health threat facing African American women is obesity, and all of the maladies that attend it. Heart disease, diabetes, high blood pressure, respiratory disorders, arthritis, and even some cancers are all ailments that being obese (weighing 20 percent or more over one's ideal body weight) puts you at risk for, according to the National Institutes of Health (NIH).

As with a lot of problems afflicting black women, we're not the only ones with a weight problem, we've just got it worse than everyone else. The irony is that despite a very real disparity between the quality of healthcare we receive and the quality received by other groups, the biggest threat we face is the one we have the most control over. Sedentary lifestyles and "diets of poverty" that are high in fat and low in fruits and vegetables (fried chicken, cheese fries, pastries) are partly to blame, says NIH. Despite the stereotype that blacks are athletic, half of our men and 67 percent of our women participate in little or no leisure-time physical activity at all, according to the third National Health and Nutrition Examination survey.

The "big, beautiful woman" image that we sisters proudly adopt is also to blame, says Patricia Davidson, M.D., a Washington, DC-area cardiologist. Magazines, advertisements, and other media images that promote the virtues of voluptuousness are not simply about loving ourselves the way that we are despite what society tells us about beauty. They are in fact destructive, because they feed into the denial that many black women have about their weight problem, says Davidson. To her and the other health care professionals who addressed the conference, actress/comedienne Mo'Nique's book, *Skinny Women Are Evil* (Atria Books, $23), is no joke. (See chapter 24 for how Mo'Nique has since changed her lifestyle.)

But are most black women really in denial about the need to slim down? Not according to the 2003 Nia Enterprises Health Survey, which was conducted in conjunction with BWHI, with top-line results unveiled at the colloquium. Nearly two-thirds of the respondents said their biggest health concern was one of the following: weight, diet/nutrition, or fitness. Of these,

34 percent cited weight, 17 percent cited diet and nutrition, and 10 percent cited fitness. (More than 1000 women participated in the survey, nearly all of them members of NiaOnline's Consumer Advisory Panel.)

Recognizing that there's a problem and correcting it are two different things. Without the support of friends, family, and community, most black women will not be successful in their battle with the bulge, said experts at the colloquium. Changes in diet, activity, and lifestyle don't happen in a vacuum. Solutions suggested at the meeting that are more likely to be effective include self-help groups that focus on healthy cooking, eating, and fitness, and which also rely on the buddy system for support.

What also needs to improve is the "superwoman" attitude that leads us to neglect our own well-being because we claim to be too busy taking care of others. After all, how many people do we know whose mothers didn't live long enough to finish taking care of them? Marilyn Hughes Gaston, M.D., who is a former U.S. assistant surgeon general and BWHI board member, likens the risks associated with being "superwoman" to the warning all airplane passengers get before a flight takes off. In the event of a change in cabin pressure, you are advised to put the air mask on yourself before assisting your child with his or her mask. "Otherwise, you may become unconscious," she describes. "We (black women) are unconscious now because we're so busy taking care of everyone else."

23

A Diet Plan

DESIGNED FOR SISTERS

In this chapter, NiaOnline asks physician Robert S. Beale important questions about diet and finds out about a diet plan designed specifically for sisters.

According to the American Obesity Association, 78 percent of African American women are overweight—the highest rate of any racial or ethnic group. Robert S. Beale Jr., M.D., a Washington, DC, bariatric physician, says he has treated thousands of overweight sisters since opening his practice in 1977.

Many have been unable to lose weight no matter how religiously they adhere to their diet and exercise programs, he says. Dr. Beale now believes that the legacy of slavery has changed the metabolism of many black Americans, making weight loss especially difficult.

Based on his clinical observations, Dr. Beale has devised

a sisters-only weight-loss method explained in the book *The Black Diet Doctor's Solution for Black Women.* While his theories have not been proved scientifically, we think his approach is worth considering (see more at www.thedietsolutions.com).

Curious? Read on.

Q: **You claim that the reason many sisters have trouble losing weight is that their metabolism has been altered by slavery. What exactly do you mean?**

A: Most of us are the descendants of slaves, either West Indian or American. We were bred to do a lot of work and not need a lot of food. Our great-great-great-grandmothers could work in the field all day on a pig's tail and still maintain their body size. Therefore, you may not be able to go to a gym and force your body to burn a lot of fat.

Q: **You claim that some black women must take different steps than other women to lose weight successfully.**

A: The notion that exercise and a healthy diet can cause all black women to lose a significant amount of weight is fallacious. Even when following a proper diet—such as eating whole-grain cereals, fruits, and vegetables and baking your chicken thighs and taking the skins off—many black American women are still unlikely to lose weight.

Q: **Why do you state that Atkins, low-carb, and other popular diets may not work for us?**

A: In general, black women with 30 or more pounds to lose who follow Atkins will lose a few pounds at first, and then the weight will pile back on. They also run the risk of increasing their cholesterol and triglycerides, a type of fat found in the blood. A lot of low-carb diets do not have enough fruits and vegetables. It's bad for the heart, liver, and kidneys to eat that much protein and fat without carbohydrates.

Q: How do you characterize your weight-loss program?

A: I've developed four different plans depending on the person's size. They are designed to get weight off *now* by forcing the body to live partly on food and partly on stored fat. Once you get to the weight that you want to be, you switch to a healthy eating plan, which will prevent you from making new fat.

Q: What does each plan require, and what results can a woman expect?

A: Each provides a list of healthy foods that, through trial and error, we've found will [help you] lose weight; and if you don't eat them, you *may* not lose weight. If the food is on the list, you can have it; if it's not, you can't. We don't recommend eating as little as possible—some of our plans for larger ladies say not to restrict the amounts. The average overweight woman will lose two to three pounds a week, eight to nine pounds a month.

Q: You say this diet isn't low-carb, yet I notice that your food lists contain certain fruits and vegetables but omit healthy starches like brown rice and beans.

A: For weight reduction, I have found that starches—including rice, pasta, potatoes, beans, bread, and crackers—are not necessary to maintain good health. In fact, they slow the rate of weight loss. Fruits and vegetables are absolutely necessary for energy and to maintain good health.

Q: **Why do you differentiate between weight loss and weight maintenance?**

A: You have to eat a certain way to get weight off and another way to keep it off. When you're losing, you're living partially on food and partially on stored fat, which is not normal. To maintain, you live totally on food but follow a strategy to avoid manufacturing new fat.

Q: **On your program, exercise seems to take a backseat to dietary changes.**

A: The larger the person, the more dangerous exercise is. The smaller the person, the more important it is. We're concerned about larger people hurting themselves—their knees, ankles, and back and getting pulled muscles—and a lot of exercise may be bad for their heart. As [a larger person] gets smaller, we increase exercise to firm and tone and help maintain the weight loss.

Q: **You've spoken about weight maintenance, but I notice you don't write much about it in the book—or portion sizes, or healthy cooking techniques. You say eat what you wish "within reason." Why don't you provide more in-depth advice in these areas that are so vital to maintaining a healthy weight?**

A: People eat what they want most of the time. You can't give them hard-and-fast rules. And I don't think it's useful to provide long lists of foods and calories and fat grams and tell people to measure them out every day. I say eat "within reason." That means don't make yourself sick. If you have high cholesterol, you can't eat french fries all day.

To gain a pound of fat, you have to eat 3,475 extra calories. You can't eat that in a day, so you can't gain a pound in a day—it's even hard in a week. Once people weigh what they wish, we tell them to weigh themselves every morning. If they've picked up weight that day, it's mostly water but also some fat. For that day, they should go back on the weight-loss program. They will probably need to do this for one or two days each week.

Note: *As with all weight-loss programs, experts see things differently. Nutritionist Goulda Downer, Ph.D., R.D, president of Metroplex Health and Nutrition Services in Washington, DC, weighs in on Dr. Beale's approach:*

"This is a high-protein, semistarvation diet," she says. "It includes carbohydrates in the form of fruits and vegetables but is missing grains, bread, and the B-complex nutrients (thiamine, riboflavin, niacin, and so on) found in them that release energy from the foods we eat.

"It's also low in fats, which our bodies need as part of a balanced, wholesome, and tasty plan. Fats keep us fuller for a longer period of time so that we are not constantly hungry, which is counterproductive to most eating plans.

"We should not be vilifying any food item or food group. All foods can fit. As for portion control, it is the foundation for any long-term solution. That way, people do not feel deprived. The question to ask is, can I eat like this for the rest of my life? And while I wish this approach offered information about portion control or healthy ways to prepare food, I like that it offers programs for women of different sizes.

"I don't know that I agree with the assertion that slavery has changed our metabolism," Downer continues. "It might have changed our metabolism. But we need to take responsibility for what we put in our mouths today. And black women need so much help in achieving a healthy weight that I wish this program had been documented scientifically so we could prove it works."

24

Q&A: Comedian Mo'Nique on Diet *and* Exercise

Full-figured comedienne Mo'Nique loves to prove haters wrong, especially those who assume that big girls can't look just as good and move just as well as their skinny counterparts. Who could forget her showstopping performance of Beyoncé's "Crazy in Love" dance routine at the 2004 BET Awards? In this chapter, journalist, television writer, and producer Sherri A. McGee asks Mo'Nique questions about dieting. Sherri McGee is the coauthor, with Mo'Nique, of the New York Times *bestselling book* Skinny Women Are Evil: Notes of a Big Girl in a Small-Minded World. *She also served as an assistant and writer on the UPN comedy* The Parkers *and cowrote the film* Hair Show.

Mo'Nique made a memorable impression at the 2004 BET Awards, but whether or not she still thinks "skinny women are evil," the funny girl has made some changes in her lifestyle, and it shows. In early 2005, NiaOnline caught up with the shapely Queen of Comedy to find out what's behind her new glow and streamlined good looks. In this wide-ranging Q&A, she talks about her fitness routine, her sensible approach to food, and how she maintains her healthy self-image in Tinseltown.

Q: You always look beautiful, but lately there seems to be less of you. What have you done to lose so much weight?

A: This is probably gonna sound crazy, but I'm still 250 pounds. I've only lost about ten pounds, but what I've lost is a lot of inches.

Q: Really? How did you do that?

A: A girlfriend was at my home, and she had this glow. I asked her what she was doing, and she told me she'd been walking on the beach to clear her mind. So I started walking with her. We laughed, cried, and encouraged each other. After three months, we were up to fifteen miles a day. Walking allowed me to be honest with myself. It was just space, air, and one foot in front of the other.

Q: So losing weight wasn't a conscious decision, but it became a wonderful one.

A: Definitely, and I love the results.

Q: Did you see results immediately?

A: Baby, yes! My pants started falling off. My waist got thinner, and my behind got tighter. Sex is great too. I'm doing things I never have before. And my spirit changed. I became more introspective and focused. Everyone in Los Angeles looks good, and I wanted to look good too.

Q: Would you ever consider plastic surgery?

A: Hell, no! This town is full of folks who've cut, sewed, tucked, and plucked themselves beyond recognition. I'm OK with what God gave me, despite the fact that a doctor once told me I needed to have [gastric bypass] surgery because I had the fat gene. There's no going back after that. I got up and got the hell out of there quick. Everyone is looking for the quick fix, and when they get it, their heads are too big for their bodies. I'm proud of what I've achieved—naturally.

Q: What's your workout routine now?

A: I still walk. But I also joined a gym. I lift light weights, do leg lifts, and work out on the Lifestride [treadmill] machine. My advice to big girls: Don't start in a high-impact aerobics class—you'll kill yourself. Take it slow. Walk. Get back in touch with your beautiful self!

Q: How have your eating habits changed?

A: Where I'm from in Baltimore, there's a soul food restaurant on every corner. In L.A., I have to drive to get to the good ones because there aren't many in my neighborhood. I've discovered great restaurants and new dishes that are healthy *and* taste good.

Q: Do you have any health issues?

A: I have high blood pressure, and I'm working to get it under control. Other than that, I've always been told by physicians that I'm healthy.

Q: **Do you follow a special diet?**

A: Not really. I pretty much eat what I want, but I'll usually do a Caesar salad with chicken or shrimp. I eat a lot of baked chicken, and I love buffalo wings with a salad. I've also discovered apples. They'll keep you moving, if you know what I mean. I've also learned not to eat heavy at night and now keep healthier snacks—like applesauce and fruit cups—in the refrigerator.

Q: **Do you have a sweet tooth?**

A: Thankfully, no. But every now and then, if I feel like having a piece of that sock-it-to-me cake, I'll have it. I just don't have all of it. I've also increased my water intake, but drinking water is something I constantly have to work at.

Q: **What do you think of the portions served in restaurants these days?**

A: I'm all for folks getting their money's worth, but nowadays it's just too much food—even for big girls. Everyone's toting doggie bags home. Pork chops taste great, but you can't eat 'em every night, and trust me, there was a time when I ate whatever I wanted at all hours of the night. Our bodies can't sustain that. The food industry thrives on keeping us stuffed.

Q: **What happened to the days when your mom prepared dinner every evening?**

A: My mother still has dinner on the table by six every evening. Whenever I'm home or near a kitchen, I'll make dinner. I'm also developing a cookbook.

Q: What kind of cookbook will it be?

A: It's called "No Damn Substitutes," and it will feature complete meals that are healthy *and* taste good, as only a big girl can bring it to you!

25

The Challenge *of the* Forties

MAKING WELLNESS A PRIORITY

Cheryl Mayberry McKissack is the founder, president, and chief executive officer of NiaOnline. Previously, Mayberry McKissack served as senior vice president and general manager of worldwide sales and marketing for Open Port Technology. She was responsible for the direction and implementation of all sales, marketing, product management, and business development/strategic alliances. Before joining Open Port, Mayberry McKissack was vice president of sales/Americas for 3Com Corporation (formerly U.S. Robotics), where she was one of the founders of its Network Systems Division. She also enjoyed a fourteen-year career with IBM in various sales and marketing management positions. Mayberry McKissack has a bachelor's degree in political science from Seattle University and an MBA from the Kellogg School of Management at Northwestern University, where she was recently named adjunct professor of entrpreneurship. Here, she talks about the health challenges that so many black women face, her personal lifestyle goals, and the changes she's embracing to choose wellness and make it a top priority in her life.

I must admit that as a black woman in my forties, I have been extremely blessed with relatively good health. Other than a recurring problem with fibroids, a scare several years ago with a benign tumor, and some minor issues, I have been given wellness without having made a conscious decision to choose it. But the idea of choosing wellness is important, and I have been consistently reminded of it as I've witnessed friends and loved ones struggle to deal with health issues that have taken away their ability to make this choice. I am reminded of what happens to a life when the opportunity to choose is taken away whenever I think about the untimely passing of my father.

My father was a healthy man in his early fifties when illness struck suddenly and swiftly. Over the next three years, he went from living an active life to being on kidney dialysis three days a week to ultimately dying of a heart attack from treatment complications. I remember asking my father my standard question shortly before his death: "How are you doing?" Instead of saying his usual, "I am doing OK," Dad's reply was quite different this time.

"Baby, I am not really living; I just exist, taking up space," he said. "My life today consists of dialysis three times a week, resting and recovering from the treatments the rest of the time, and maybe for 30 minutes a week I will feel OK, not great! My health does not allow me to work, to travel, to have friends, or to enjoy my family; it just allows me to exist." I remember feeling very distressed after speaking to my father, and shortly after this conversation, he passed away. He was just fifty-six years old.

Coming to Terms With Our Own Health Challenges

Over the last three years, I have personally witnessed several of my friends in their forties struggle with life-threatening illnesses and come face-to-face with their own mortality. One of my dear friends is dealing with this battle today. I admire her spirit and tenacity, and I continue to be amazed how, in the midst of her struggles, she chooses wellness every day. She demonstrates daily how an individual can use her intellectual and spiritual strengths to fight an illness that has changed her life forever.

I am sure that many people have experienced the loss of a loved one or faced the reality of how illness can change your life. So I ask the question: Why don't we choose wellness and take better care of ourselves, since we all know the alternative? The health statistics for African Americans are startling and scary and make a strong argument for focusing on wellness. Consider these recent health statistics:

- African Americans have higher rates of colorectal cancer than any other racial or ethnic group in the United States, according to the Black Women's Health Imperative.
- As the Black Women's Health Imperative also points out, African Americans are four times more likely than white Americans to develop kidney failure.
- The prevalence of high blood pressure in African Americans is the highest in the world, according to the American Stroke Association.

- On average, black Americans are twice as likely as white Americans of similar age to have diabetes, according to the National Diabetes Information Clearinghouse.

If we look specifically at black women, the statistics tell an even more disturbing story:

- With a life expectancy of 76 years, African American women live, on average, four years less than white women, according to the Centers for Disease Control and Prevention (CDC).
- In a study by the University of Chicago, black women in the United States under the age of 35 had a 50 percent greater risk than white women of developing breast cancer.
- Black women make up nearly two-thirds of all HIV-positive women in the United States, according to Black Women's Health Imperative.

Embracing the Decision to Choose Wellness

These headlines and statistics should inspire all of us to schedule an appointment with our doctor for a full physical, but it is unlikely that most of us will do so. Recently, however, while facing another rapidly approaching birthday, I decided to take stock of my own health. Although I have never smoked or used drugs, I knew there were many things that I could be doing to improve my overall well-being. To begin my journey, I asked myself the question, "What does choosing wellness mean to me?" I came up with a three-part answer:

1. Choosing wellness means acknowledging that wellness is not just given to us and that, even though there is no guarantee that we will remain healthy, there are steps all of us can take to assist the process.

2. Choosing wellness means realizing that we can have it all, just not all the time. This doesn't mean drinking wheatgrass every day; but we must be willing to give up some of our vices in order to progress along the path of wellness.

3. Choosing wellness means accepting that none of the success that any of us will achieve will be greater than wellness and good health. Wellness is the essential ingredient in our enjoyment of the success that we strive to achieve. Without a healthy body, mind, and spirit, nothing else matters.

So why do black women have some of the highest rates of disease in so many categories? My own theory stems from the belief that we have not learned the importance of taking care of ourselves first so that we can be the best we can be for ourselves and our loved ones. According to the CDC, 55 percent of African American women are physically inactive, and 78 percent are classified as overweight or obese. Yet how many times have we heard another sister say, or even remarked ourselves, "I would work out in the morning, but I can't sweat out my hair"? A 2004 NiaOnline survey of black women discovered that those polled were more likely to give up exercise in their daily lives than give up good grooming. We must start to focus on what is going on inside instead of placing so much importance on how we look on the outside.

Additionally, we must accept that while fitness is important, choosing wellness is not synonymous with slimming down. The true meaning of wellness is a balance of physical, mental, and spiritual health that covers all of the key areas—not just weight.

So how do you build a plan for yourself to choose wellness?

Everyone is different, and each of us must develop a realistic objective and regimen that we can live with. But I would like to share with you my program for choosing wellness, because I think you may find that some aspects apply to your own life. I decided that the foundation of my plan would consist of three elements:

1. *Education:* I decided to find out what types of health information were available, how to access that information, and which tools existed to keep me updated on a regular basis. The internet is a terrific resource for researching questions and obtaining an enormous range of information. I discovered that organizations like the American Heart Association offer an abundance of information, along with programs tailored to the needs of African American women and their families. In the Resource Guide at the end of this book, you will see a listing of other organizations that offer useful information about your health and that of your family.

2. *Environment:* I realized that I had to create the optimal physical, mental, and spiritual environment to help me be the best that I can be. This included letting go of negative energy and influences and replacing them with positive, spiritual energy and activities that would allow me to focus on this lifetime quest of choosing wellness. For instance, I have decided to surround myself with positive people instead of those who focus on the negative aspects of life.

3. *Advocacy:* I made it a priority to promote wellness among African American women and their households. NiaOnline had previously partnered with the Black Women's Health Imperative to conduct a study

about health issues facing African American women. I decided going forward that my advocacy efforts would use technology and the NiaOnline network of black households, and also include partnerships with other organizations that were committed to improving the health of those households. Our focus has included spreading the word about the dangers of not making an informed decision to choose wellness and simply taking the chance that it will choose you. The writing and promotion of this book is a critical step in our journey to inform and educate black women, as well as to encourage you to choose wellness.

Applying Life Lessons

Once I had established the foundation of the overall plan, I decided to make it more personal by evaluating my own lifestyle and deciding how I could apply my three-point plan to my own wellness challenges. What specific activities did I include in my own list of personal goals?

I decided to conduct a self-assessment and be honest about what I need to do to be at my personal best.

1. I had to come to terms with certain truths about my current habits:
   - Lattes in the morning are not a substitute for a breakfast meal.
   - Staying busy all day and eating my main meal late in the evening is not the best way to balance my dietary intake. Skipping meals can lead to overeating later in the day, say dieticians.
   - Strength training is great, but my body type and age also require cardio activity several times a week.

- Achieving balance between the professional and personal in my own life is a critical part of creating overall wellness—and is the subject of the previous book in the Nia Guide for Black Women series: *Balancing Work and Life.*

2. I made an appointment to have a full physical. It was important that I look at the diseases that are part of my family history, such as diabetes, and review my own health status.

3. I revamped my exercise program and increased my physical activity, establishing a workout schedule of at least three or four times a week. I also added variety to my fitness regimen by incorporating running, Pilates, and strength training.

4. I focused on my mental and spiritual needs in addition to my physical health. I am once again attending church regularly, and the weekly Pilates session helps me to relieve stress.

5. I entered a cleansing program to learn more about the way my body functions and to improve my eating habits.

6. I incorporated a variety of all-natural vitamins and minerals into my daily dietary program.

I am happy to report that I have completed my cleansing program, lost 13 pounds, and established a regular exercise program. I am also contributing to my mental and physical health by periodically evaluating my environment for negative influences. I have expanded my advocacy through outreach with friends and family, and my beloved 71-year-old mother has started an exercise program for the first time in her life and is up to 45 minutes a day on her treadmill!

I realize that this is only the beginning of my journey, and I must commit to making these changes a lifetime program and a top priority in my life. To truly choose wellness requires daily focus and determination. I understand that life holds no guarantee, but I also believe that there is tremendous value in taking responsibility for your health and in choosing wellness as a vital part of your everyday life.

26

The Black Women's Health Imperative

on WALKING FOR WELLNESS

and 4 STEPS TO A SLIMMER YOU

Walking is one of the easiest, cheapest, safest, and most effective ways to exercise. It's also a great way to work your heart muscle; reduce the risks of health problems including heart disease, stroke, diabetes, and Alzheimer's disease; relieve stress; shed some pounds; and enjoy Mother Earth. All those benefits without treks to the gym, expensive equipment, or sweating out your 'do.

The Black Women's Health Imperative launched its Walking for Wellness program several years ago, encouraging women to walk at least 10,000 steps daily or three 30-minute walking sessions weekly. Impressed by its practical and flexible approach, we asked them to share the program with our readers. Whether you form a walking group for sister-support or make a solo commitment to walk the path to success, the Walking for Wellness program can show you how it's done. Get ready!

Walking for Wellness Boot Camp

You probably think you know all there is to know about walking. You started your training as a toddler. Since then, you've been doing it daily on a professional level, right? Well, slow your stroll. There are a few dos and don'ts that you'll need to master. And even though walking is a free activity, there are a few items that you'll need to invest in for this program, too. Before you know it, you'll graduate from a beginner to an advanced Walker for Wellness toward the ultimate goal of 10,000 daily steps.

In addition to the information you find here, enroll in the free online version of the Black Women's Health Imperative's Walking for Wellness program at www.blackwomenshealth.org. The Black Women's Health Imperative will take this Walking for Wellness journey with you, offering motivation, guidance, and companionship along the way. You'll receive an online log for your activity sessions; nutrition analysis and tips; behavior modification instruction and monthly feature stories; and tips about Walking for Wellness delivered directly to your email in order to keep you motivated.

Medical Precaution Tips Before You Begin

Prior to starting this or any exercise program, get a doctor's OK. Please schedule your physical today, if you haven't already.

Also, be on the lookout for these warning signs as you adjust to your new walking program.

- If you develop chest pain, excessive fatigue, dizziness, or shortness of breath while walking, stop walking immediately and seek help.
- If you develop a side stitch or leg cramp while walking, stop walking and stretch.
- Try to avoid any form of exercise immediately after eating, which can make you uncomfortable while walking.
- Drink plenty of fluids to avoid dehydration.
- Don't push yourself too hard, especially as you adjust to this new walking routine.

Shoe Smarts

Don't waste money on expensive, celebrity-endorsed walking shoes. Try to find the best sale on the most comfortable pair of walking shoes that you can find. Here are some general guidelines for selecting your shoes:

- The top or upper part of the shoes should be made of leather, canvas, or nylon. These materials allow your feet to breathe by allowing air to circulate. Remember, your feet become hot and sweaty from walking.
- The shoes should have a durable but soft sole that cushions your feet. They should be padded at the heel and under the ball of the foot to protect your feet from hard surfaces such as city streets and sidewalks.
- The shoes should support both the heel and the arch. They should fit snugly around the widest part of your feet. The shoes should have between a quarter- and a half-inch of space between your longest toe and the tip of the shoe. Look for shoes with a squared-off toe area

or "toe box," which is very comfortable for most fitness walkers.

- Look for shoes that are tilted at the toe (it helps with the heel-to-toe walking motion), raised at the heel (it reduces the risk of tendon strain), and relatively lightweight (it'll help you move quicker).
- When you shop for walking shoes, test them with the socks you'll wear while exercising.
- Shop in the evening or after you've taken a brisk walk. Feet tend to swell during the course of the day and during exercise. You want to purchase shoes that'll fit your feet at their biggest!

Pedometer Readings

Next to your walking shoes, a pedometer is the most important tool you'll purchase for the Walking for Wellness program. Why do you need one? It'll keep you motivated and aware of your daily fitness goal of 10,000 steps. How does it work? A pedometer multiplies the number of steps you take by the stride length you enter and then divides that number by 5,280 (the number of feet in a mile). Therefore, if you want your distance measurement to be accurate, it is important to enter an accurate stride length (follow the directions on your pedometer).

We recommend that you wear a pedometer for a week after purchasing it. Put it on as soon as you wake in the morning and leave it on for the duration of the day. This practice week will give you a good indication of how many steps you average on a typical day. Based on your test-week performance, the goal of 10,000 daily steps might seem too challenging. Don't worry. You'll build on your daily steps, adding intensity and time to your workouts gradually.

Pick Your Plan

Here are four walking plans that'll help you fit fitness into your hectic schedule and add more steps to your day.

Plan 1: Maximize the Minimum

Who it's for: The woman who rarely has a free minute during a typical day.

Your goal: Log 2,000-4,000 steps daily or 30 minutes of exercise 5 days a week. To reach this goal, you must make an effort to be as active as possible, even on your hectic days.

How to do it: Maximize your weekends (or the days you have a less rigid schedule) and make do on the rest.

Plan 1: Your Walking Week	
Sunday	25 minutes brisk walking; stretching
Monday	Off
Tuesday	Morning: 15 minutes brisk walking; stretching Evening: stretching
Wednesday	Morning: 10 minutes brisk walking; stretching Lunch: 20 minutes brisk walking; stretching
Thursday	Off
Friday	15 minutes brisk walking; stretching
Saturday	45 minutes brisk walking; stretching

Stretching: Always stretch after your walks. It'll increase your flexibility, improve your walking form, and help prevent injury.

Strength component: Learn several quick, total-body strength exercises you can do anywhere. Try squats and abdominal crunches. Or get some elastic exercise bands and learn how to do basic strength exercises with them.

Tips:

- Pack your exercise into short, high-intensity efforts. At least three days of the week focus on fast walking, even if it's just for 10-15 minutes.
- Make walking activities a part of things you do already. Turn transit time into exercise: walk or bike to work, get off the subway or the bus a stop early or walk the kids to school. Also, focus on fidgeting: Pace while talking on the phone or stroll the long hallways in airport terminals while waiting for a flight.
- Try early morning walks. Some of the busiest people find exercising early in the morning to be effective and rewarding. (Be sure to try it for a couple of weeks so your body clock has time to adjust before passing judgment.)
- Find just a few more holes in your week to walk. Look for short demands on your time that aren't absolutely critical: Can you forgo carpool duty once in a while, skip a meeting now and then, or pass on one of your daily chats with your sister?

The Results: You'll have increased energy, improved health and—just maybe—an iota of control over your life.

- Daily goal steps: 2,000–4,000
- Estimated calories burned per week: 1,000
- Pounds lost in a year: 14

Plan 2: Make Every Minute Count

Who it's for: The woman who doesn't have much free time, but who does have some breaks or flexibility in her day.

Your goal: Aim for at least 30 minutes of exercise six days a week.

How to do it: Make the most of your breaks by squeezing activity into multiple brief efforts.

Plan 2: Your Walking Week	
Sunday	40 minutes brisk walking; stretching
Monday	Off
Tuesday	Morning: 10 minutes brisk walking; stretching Evening: 15 minutes brisk walking; upper body toning; stretching
Wednesday	Morning: 10 minutes brisk walking; stretching Lunch: 10 minutes brisk walking; stretching
Thursday	Morning: 15 minutes brisk walking; stretching Lunch: 15 minutes brisk walking; stretching
Friday	Off
Saturday	Morning: 20 minutes brisk walking; stretching Evening: 10 minutes brisk walking; upper and lower body toning; stretching

Stretching: Always stretch after your walks. It'll increase your flexibility, improve walking form, and help prevent injury.

Strength component: Get some three- and five-pound dumbbells and learn six to eight simple strength-training exercises. Separate them into two routines of 10 minutes each: curls, presses, and rows for the upper body; squats, lunges, and step-ups for the lower body.

Tips:

- Look for small breaks between other activities during the day. Remember that even 10 minutes is enough to count.
- Plan on more than one workout a day. Your lifestyle is better suited to two or three short walks than one long one.
- Keep walking gear handy. Walking shoes, a water bottle, a towel, and a clean shirt in your car or desk drawer can make an ever-ready fitness center.

- You don't always have to break a sweat. With that in mind, consider easier brief walks crammed in between meetings or while waiting for a child to finish a piano lesson. Save the more taxing efforts for when a shower is within easy access.

The results: Improved health and a stable, healthy weight, plus you'll feel a sense of accomplishment as you make progress.
- Daily goal steps: 4,000–6,000 steps
- Estimated calories burned per week: 1,200
- Pounds lost in a year: 18

Plan 3: Stick With Structure

Who it's for: The woman who has some time for exercise, but who also has very structured days with few breaks.

Your goal: Adhere to a structured seven-day-a-week program. Average 30 minutes most days and up to 40 minutes or more two or three days of the week.

How to do it: Build regular, formal exercise time into your weekly schedule and treat it as seriously as you would any other commitment.

Plan 3: Your Walking Week	
Sunday	50 minutes (longer when you can); stretching
Monday	20 minutes fast walking; stretching
Tuesday	15 minutes fast walking; 25 minutes strength training; stretching
Wednesday	35 minutes brisk walking
Thursday	15 minutes brisk walking; stretching
Friday	25 minutes fast walking; stretching
Saturday	40 minutes brisk walking; 25 minutes strength training; stretching

Stretching: Always stretch after your walks. It'll increase your flexibility, improve walking form and help prevent injury.

Strength component: Find a regular place for strength training, whether it's a health club, a local YMCA, a fitness center at work, or even a weight room in your basement. Learn a total-body conditioning program that you can complete in roughly 25 minutes; schedule two or three sessions a week.

Tips:

- Emphasize high intensity when time is tight. On your busiest days, focus on briefer, faster walks.
- Schedule your workouts on a weekly calendar. This ensures you'll use the breaks you do have, plus it locks in workout time.
- Make specific appointments to work out with others. Agree on how long and how far you'll walk ahead of time and stick to it.
- Use your support network. Have your spouse pitch in with the housework so you can walk.

The results: Improved fitness and muscle tone, and measurable progress toward weight loss. What's more, you'll begin to feel (and look) like an athlete.

- Daily goal steps: 6,000–8,000 steps
- Estimated calories burned per week: 1,500
- Pounds lost in a year: 22

Plan 4: Go All Out!

Who it's for: The woman who has some available time in the day and some breaks or flexibility in her schedule.

Your goal: Follow a regular, seven-day schedule. Mix longer, slower-paced walks with shorter, faster walks.

How to do it: Create formal opportunities to exercise (such as meeting a friend for a regular walk) and learn to make exercise a part of your lifestyle.

Plan 4: Your Walking Week	
Sunday	60 minutes fast walking; stretching
Monday	20 minutes fast walking; stretching
Tuesday	40 minutes fast walking; stretching
Wednesday	20 minutes brisk walking; 30 minutes yoga or stretching
Thursday	Morning: 25 minutes easy walking; stretching Evening: 20 minutes fast walking; stretching
Friday	15 minutes fast walking; stretching
Saturday	30 minutes fast walking; 40 minutes strength training; stretching

Stretching: Always stretch after your walks. It'll increase your flexibility, improve walking form, and help prevent injury.

Strength component: Plan on attending a 30- to 45-minute strength class two days per week, or schedule a regular time each week to work out with friends or a personal trainer. For a change of pace, consider a yoga or a tai chi class.

Tips:

- Build in variety. Plan varied distances and speed to keep your walking interesting; try to average at least 40 minutes of exercise per day.
- Join a walking club. Commit to one or two workouts a week. Promise to bring the water bottles to make sure you don't skip practice.
- Tell family and friends exercise is a priority. Ask them to be supportive of your workout schedule.
- Examine your week for time better spent. You may want to consider losing a television program (or hop on the

treadmill during it) or an unnecessary obligation each week.

The results: Greatly improved aerobic conditioning and muscular strength. Over time, you'll notice not just weight loss, but firmer, shapelier muscles and a greater ability to handle day-to-day tasks.

- Daily Goal Steps: 8,000–10,000
- Estimated calories burned per week: 1,900
- Pounds lost in a year: 28

Stretching Tips

If you're tired of feeling tight (your knees crack when you rise too quickly) or if you want to tie your shoelaces with ease (without having to sit down), it's important to add stretching into your new Walking for Wellness routine.

Flexibility (how well your joints and muscles move through a range of motion) decreases with age, inactivity, or improperly performed exercise. Stretching exercises will help you with these issues, as well as walking form and injury prevention. They are also great ways to relieve stress.

We recommend that you take just 10 minutes to stretch after your 5-minute walking warm-up and after each exercise session to help you cool-down. Perform each stretch slowly and smoothly. Do not bounce. You should feel a gentle pull or stretch in the muscle without any pain.

Also, remember to work at your own pace. Don't compare your stretches to a dance diva's dynamics. Simply work on getting the best stretch that your body can achieve. You'll notice gradual improvements as you do the movements regularly.

Wait until after you've warmed up your body or until after your workout to stretch. You risk straining or pulling a muscle if you do it while the body is cold. Remember, stretching should feel good. When you stretch, extend to the point of tension and hold for 15 to 20 seconds. Always stretch slowly with a relaxed, smooth movement. Do not hold your breath. Slow, steady breathing will help muscles relax.

Here's the 411 on stretching. Include these easy moves in your Walking for Wellness program to keep you flexible, especially when time is tight.

The Butterfly

Goal: To stretch the inner thigh muscles
Repetitions: 4 times, hold for 8 counts

1. Sit down on the floor with the soles of your feet touching each other.
2. Place your elbows on the area where your legs fold (behind the knee).
3. Place slight pressure from your elbows down on your legs, enough to allow for a stretch.
4. Hold for eight counts.
5. Repeat four times.
6. Try to keep your back straight. You may have a tendency to bend forward slightly, but try not to slump over.
7. Keep stomach tucked in and remember to breathe.

Arm Stretch

Goal: To stretch out arms and back
Repetitions: 2 times, hold for 8 counts

1. Stand with your feet firmly on the ground, parallel and about 12 inches apart.
2. Keep your back straight and stomach tucked in.

3. Standing in front of a doorway, place your arms fully extended behind you and hold the frame with the tips of your fingers.
4. Pull away from the doorway slightly, allowing for your arms and back to feel the stretch.
5. Hold this position for about 8 counts.
6. Repeat twice.

Side Stretch

Goal: To stretch trunk

Repetitions: 5 times on each side, hold for 5 counts

1. Stand with your feet firmly on the ground, parallel and about 12 inches apart.
2. Keep your back straight and stomach tucked in.
3. Clasp hands together and raise your arms above your head (some people may find it easier to keep one hand on their waist).
4. Bend trunk slowly to the right (this should take about 5 counts to be into position).
5. Hold this position for 5 counts.
6. Return to your upright position in 5 counts.
7. Do the same movement to the left side.
8. Repeat 5 times on each side.

Leg Stretch

Goal: To relax hamstring muscles

Repetitions: 1 time on each side, hold for 8 counts

- While sitting on the floor, extend your left leg in front of you while keeping the right leg bent, with the right knee touching the floor and the sole of the right foot against the left knee.

- Point the left foot's toes upward, and keep the back of the left heel flat on the ground.
- With your back straight, reach toward your toes as far as you can without straining.
- Hold for a count of 8.
- Repeat on the other side.

Squats

Goal: Stretch and tone the thighs and rear (gluteal) muscles
Repetitions: 2 times, hold for 8 counts

- Keep your back straight and stomach tucked in.
- With your toes pointing slightly outward, separate your feet about 18 inches.
- Slowly bend your legs enough to lower your body 6 inches to a foot (don't stick out your butt).
- Hold for 8 counts, then stand up slowly.
- Repeat.

Calf Stretch

Goal: To stretch heel and Achilles tendon and prevent injuries
Repetitions: 1 time on each side, hold for 10 counts

1. Use wall for balance, if needed.
2. Stand with right foot in front, with knee bent.
3. Place hands against wall or on waist, if you choose not to use a wall.
4. Keeping left leg straight, lean forward over bent knee. Keep body low and both feet on the ground.
5. Hold stretch for count of 10. (You should feel a tugging in the calf on the left leg.)
6. Repeat on the other side.

Bend Over

Goal: To relax after your series of stretches
Repetitions: 1 time, hold for 10 counts

1. Bend over slowly with your knees slightly bent.
2. Keep your chin slightly tucked in.
3. Feel like your body is hanging loosely. This position should help relax your back, and shoulders, and your neck. It should not cause any straining. Your head should feel heavy, completely relaxed, and loose.
4. Feel yourself deep breathing.
5. Stay in this position for at least ten seconds.
6. Slowly raise your body to the standing position.

The Stork

Goal: To stretch out the quadriceps (the large thigh muscles)
Repetitions: 1 time on each side, hold for 20 counts

1. Keep your back straight and your stomach tucked in.
2. Rest your hand on a chair or a wall for balance, if necessary.
3. Stand on your right foot. Bend the left foot back at the knee and grasp toes with your right hand.
4. Pull left foot back and up gently until you feel your thigh stretching.
5. Hold for 20 seconds and repeat on other side.

Fitness Log

Create an activities log online on the Black Women's Health Imperative Website, www.blackwomenshealth.org. This will help you to measure your physical progress and to document your feelings about the spiritual and psychological benefits you have experienced as a result of your commitment to personal wellness.

You can also photocopy the fitness worksheet in the next chapter and use the photocopies as handy tools to keep progress of your goals and successes.

Safety Tips

Your safety is a top priority. It's always important to be on guard, especially when walking alone. Be on the lookout for strange people and unleashed dogs. Follow these simple safety rules:

- Walk with a friend, if possible. There is safety in numbers.
- Don't walk at night. Always walk in well-lit areas.
- Remove noticeable jewelry and other items that will attract unwanted attention.
- Do not wear headphones. Stay aware of your surroundings.
- Let someone know your walking route and expected return time.
- Vary your routes and walking times. You don't want strangers to learn your routine.
- Carry a cell phone. Invest in a clip or carrying case for easy access to the phone.
- Keep identification and a medical alert tag, if needed, on your person at all times. Tuck a laminated business card into your jacket pocket for an easily replaceable solution.

Mental Health

Try to check in with yourself during your walks. Ask yourself, "How am I feeling?" and "What's on my mind?" Also, if you have a walking buddy, talk to each other about the day's experiences, affirm goals, and share positive statements (e.g., poems, prayers, or something positive you intend to do for yourself).

Always remember that walking is good for the body, mind, and soul. Take a minute to connect with your inner voice, celebrate your uniqueness, and feed your spirit. Get your weekly words of wisdom and affirmation at www.blackwomenshealth. org as a part of your Walking for Wellness program.

To achieve our goals, we must stay focused on them. However, we must remember that the journey is also essential. Some would even go so far as to say the journey is more important than the destination. Honestly, we miss out on precious gifts when we concentrate so hard on the finish line that we ignore the race. We miss the sun, the breeze, the trees and flowers, not to mention connecting with our fellow runners. Besides, once we reach one finish line, there is always another. We can apply this philosophy in all areas of our life—our families, work, physical health, and spiritual development. Each day, each breath, each conversation, each action, each step is important. Be sure not to stay so focused on the outcome that you miss the important lessons along the way.

Walking for Wellness Pledge

I pledge to make Walking for Wellness a journey for life. I will walk with my head held high and with a purposeful stride. I will not allow anyone or anything to keep me from my 10,000 daily steps or three 30-minute walks per week. If I stumble off the plan, I will reach out for support at www.blackwomenshealth.org and keep on strutting. Today, I'm making a commitment to wellness of body, mind, and spirit, taking one balanced step at a time!*

*Copyright 2004 Black Women's Health Imperative. Reprinted with permission.

27

Walking *for* Wellness Worksheet

Photocopy the Walking for Wellness Worksheet and use the photocopies as handy tools to keep track of your goals and successes. At the start of each week, plan your daily activities. Be specific; note the amount of time your walking activity will take (e.g., "45 min" or "1 hr"), note your planned pace (e.g., "slow," "brisk," "fast"), and note whether or not you will do any stretching. It's OK to take a day off now and then. In those cases, just write "off". If you change your activity on the day of that activity, just correct it in the sheet. When you meet and achieve your goals, mark an "X" in the right-hand column. Soon they'll add up!

Walking Plan for Week _____

Monday	Goal:	Achieved ___
Tuesday	Goal:	Achieved ___
Wednesday	Goal:	Achieved ___
Thursday	Goal:	Achieved ___
Friday	Goal:	Achieved ___
Saturday	Goal:	Achieved ___
Sunday	Goal:	Achieved ___

Walking Plan for Week _____

Monday	Goal:	Achieved ___
Tuesday	Goal:	Achieved ___
Wednesday	Goal:	Achieved ___
Thursday	Goal:	Achieved ___
Friday	Goal:	Achieved ___
Saturday	Goal:	Achieved ___
Sunday	Goal:	Achieved ___

Walking Plan for Week _____

Monday	Goal:	Achieved ___
Tuesday	Goal:	Achieved ___
Wednesday	Goal:	Achieved ___
Thursday	Goal:	Achieved ___
Friday	Goal:	Achieved ___
Saturday	Goal:	Achieved ___
Sunday	Goal:	Achieved ___

Are You
the Right Weight?

According to the Centers for Disease Control and Prevention, body mass index (BMI) is one of the most effective tools for measuring weight status in adults. Knowing your BMI will help you understand whether you are the right weight for your height. Your BMI is calculated by the following formula:

$$BMI = \left(\frac{\text{Weight in Pounds}}{\text{(Height in inches)} \times \text{(Height in inches)}} \right) \times 703$$

For example, a woman who is 130 pounds and five feet tall has a BMI of 25, which is on the upper end of the normal range.

Below is a chart of BMI categories. However, it is important to keep in mind that women tend to have higher BMIs than men, and that BMI is only one possible indicator of your health status with regard to weight and body fat.

BMI	Weight Status
Below 18.5	Underweight
18.5 – 24.9	Normal
25.0 – 29.9	Overweight
30.0 and Above	Obese

29

WAKING UP FROM
the **Nicotine**
Nightmare:
LALAH HATHAWAY ON
QUITTING SMOKING

Smoking is a leading cause of cancer. Unfortunately,
it's also one of the most challenging addictions to beat.
In this chapter, NiaOnline shares information about
some of the health risks of smoking and talks to jazz
singer Lalah Hathaway about her fight to kick the nico-
tine habit.

Cigarettes, thankfully, no longer have much cachet in American society, but despite falling rates of usage, 46 million U.S.
adults—11 percent of them African American—still smoke, according to a 2002 report from the Centers for Disease Control
and Prevention (CDC).

The good news for black women is that we smoke slightly less
than our white counterparts (19 percent versus 22 percent, re-
spectively), according to the CDC. The bad news is that we are

actually more likely to develop smoking-related illnesses such as lung cancer, according to the American Lung Association. So for black women, kicking the habit is even more of a life-and-death decision than for others.

Among the sisters who have fought their nicotine addiction and won is jazz diva Lalah Hathaway (daughter of legendary soul singer Donny Hathaway). You may know her for her smoky, sultry voice, but you may not know that she was once a two-pack-a-day smoker. Now smoke-free in her mid-thirties, the Los Angeles–based songstress, who has worked with everyone from Mary J. Blige and Me'shell Ndegéocello to Herbie Hancock and Freddie Jackson, shares with NiaOnline her battle with nicotine addiction and how she was finally able to kick the butts.

Q: Why did you start smoking?

A: Both of my parents smoked. So did my younger sister. I started in college and was a devout Marlboro and Camel Lights smoker.

Q: How long did you do it?

A: Fifteen years, off and on. I had two significant quits. The first was at 23. I did it cold turkey. It lasted a year. The second time, I used [the antidepressant] Zyban, which made me spacey. The final time, my mother and sister gave me the [over-the-counter] NicoDerm CQ patch as Christmas gifts. This [last] time was my definitive quit.

Q: Why do you think the third time was the charm?

A: Smoking is a chemical addiction like crack, heroin, or crystal meth. The pain of wanting it is what drives you back. My health is a small part of why I quit. The primary reason was that cigarettes controlled me. I wanted to regain power over my life.

Q: **What were the immediate effects of quitting?**

A: Before, I stank. My breathing was heavy and labored. I couldn't run for long periods of time. Now, [thanks also to] my trainer, workouts are better and my lung capacity is improved.

Q: **How did quitting affect your singing?**

A: I can hit more high and low notes. There's less phlegm. And I don't get sick as often.

Q: **How has your life changed?**

A: The biggest advantage, other than saving my life, is that cigarettes don't control me. A pack of Marlboro Lights is seven dollars. I put all that money in a jar. Spiritually, I've learned that everything is a process and this is a new, day-by-day lifestyle.

Q: **What about your diet? What are you eating these days?**

A: [It's] mostly high-protein, low-carb. I love Japanese food. But I'm addicted to sugar, so that's an issue—especially when I discovered that cigarettes are cured in sugar! [Editor's note: *During the tobacco-curing process, starch in the leaves is converted to sugar, leaving cigarettes with a high sugar content.*]

Q: **Now that you've quit, are you sensitive to smoke?**

A: Extremely! I'd never date a smoker. Even as one, I wouldn't sit in smoking sections and didn't want the smell in my hair and clothes.

Q: **So, no backsliding?**

A: Just the thought of it is abhorrent to me. I needed to be able to say I did this for me. That's empowering.

PART 6

LOVING THE SKIN (AND HAIR) YOU'RE IN

30

Breakout Busters:

AVOIDING ADULT ACNE

In this chapter, NiaOnline turns to Doris J. Day, M.D., a New York—based dermatologist and author of 100 Questions and Answers About Acne *(Jones & Bartlett; $16.95), for advice on preventing adult acne.*

Acne breakouts always seem to happen at the worst times: just before a big date, the afternoon of the biggest presentation of your career, the morning of your wedding. What if you could head off a breakout before it actually came to a head on your face? "What's going on inside your body, outside in the world, and in your mind can all affect your skin," explains Doris J. Day, M.D. Knowing your body's rhythms also helps. Check out these four steps you can take to keep zits from taking you by surprise:

1. *Keep a calendar to determine a pattern of flare-ups and outbreaks.* "By the time you see a pimple, it's already

been there for some time," says Dr. Day. Which means the key is being prepared.

Because a major cause of acne is a surge in hormones right before your period, she suggests marking a calendar with a "P" for the days you are menstruating. Jot down an "F" for the days that your skin is having a flare-up. "In a couple of months you will see an "F" pattern, likely in the week before your period," explains Dr. Day, who has been practicing this method herself for years. "That is the time to be more aggressive with antiacne treatments" and preventive measures. Which brings us to . . .

2. *Don't forget to exfoliate.* "A pimple is a clogged pore, so preventive care means removing dead skin cells and stimulating collagen production for a smoother complexion," says Dr. Day. Although loofahs are too harsh for the face, topical products that contain salicylic acid are excellent and can be used once or twice a week.

Every couple of months, treat yourself to a microdermabrasion or chemical peel from a dermatologist. And don't forget that the face isn't the only place that can break out, so consider picking up a body scrub that can handle any pimples on your back, chest, or, even though you probably don't like to admit it, your butt.

3. *Be kind to your skin.* No matter how tempted you are to pop a pimple, don't. Also avoid other habits that can irritate your skin. Regardless of how instinctual it is to rest the telephone on your cheek when you're talking, to prop yourself up by leaning on your chin, or even to rub your face when you come in from the cold, resist.

"All of these things can lead to increased breakouts or dark spots and hyperpigmentation, not to mention spreading bacteria," says Dr. Day, who also does not recommend that women of color get extractions during facials. "Anything that causes inflammation or swelling can lead to dark spots in black women."

Although the abuses that we bring to our skin are a major contributor to acne, so, too, are some of our efforts to fix things. "Most of us, when we are having a breakout, tend to overdo it with cleaning, don't moisturize enough, and overscrub," Dr. Day points out. "Remember, 'squeaky-clean' is too dry [for skin]." Instead, cleanse your face gently, using your fingertips. Also, regardless of your complexion or skin type, don't skip using an SPF-infused moisturizer.

4. *Know when it's time to turn to a professional.* When nothing you do will stop the breakouts and, even worse, there are marks left behind after a pimple, it is time to go to the dermatologist. Here's how to get the most out of your visit:

Tip No. 1: Go with a list of products that you have tried and write down whether they worked or not. "Also, bring a written list of questions and jot down the answers," suggests Dr. Day.

Tip No. 2: Dr. Day says that if the dermatologist prescribes Retin-A, a popular remedy that helps skin cells mature normally so pores won't clog, moisturizing is the key to preventing the dryness and irritation that can plague many black women who use it. "So wash, moisturize, wait a few minutes, mix the Retin-A with moisturizer, apply, and then moisturize again." She also suggests asking your doctor about the milder concentrations that are now available.

Beauty Bag: Product Solutions for Acne-Free Skin

- Good Skin by Estée Lauder All Right Medicated Cleanser ($12) and Oil-Free Lotion ($17.50), created by Dr. Day, will clear skin without cleaning out your pockets.
- Neutrogena Advanced Solutions Acne Mark Fading Peel ($15; at drugstores) gently fades dark spots without irritating skin.
- Clinique Acne Solutions Body Treatment Spray ($18.50) contains salicylic acid to keep you blemish-free from head to toe.

31

Winterize Your Skin

In the next three chapters, Ayana Byrd, NiaOnline's resident beauty and hair expert, and coauthor of Hair Story: Untangling the Roots of Black Hair in America *(St. Martin's; $12.95) shares tips on keeping your skin and hair safe and healthy.*

Most of us have dry skin. Period. And during the winter, it gets worse. But you can banish dry itchy skin and "ash" if you're willing to work at it. Here are some pointers:

From the Inside Out

A great way to help beat dryness is to nourish your skin internally. Follow this advice:

- Drink at least eight glasses of water a day.
- Without overdoing it, be sure to include in your diet

monounsaturated fats (a "good" type of fat) easily found in olive and canola oils.

· Take 400 international units (IUs) of vitamin E daily (be sure to pick a brand that specifies mixed tocopherols on the label).

Tub Time

Shower or bath time can be made into a wonderfully relaxing ritual. But take care: Too much of a good thing can dry out your skin. Keeping the water too hot or soaking too long can make dry skin worse. So keep the water temperature mild, and do not linger more than 10 minutes.

That said, taking a shower or bath can also be a great way to beat winter-skin blahs:

· Arm yourself with a good loofah or body mitt and use it religiously. (Synthetic body puffs may be better than natural-fiber loofahs because they hold less bacteria and last longer, but either is fine.)

· Choose a body gel that will not dry out your skin. One great option, albeit an expensive one, is Dr. Hauschka Body Wash in Floral ($22.50). Specially made for dry, sensitive skin, the creamy concoction contains oils of rose, lilac, and jasmine.

· Once a week, treat yourself to a body scrub to remove dry dead skin and moisturize your body. There are some fantastic scrubs on the market; not enough good things can be said about Origins Ginger Body Scrub ($30). You can also make your own oatmeal or salt scrubs. Whether you use a store-bought variety or make your own scrub, apply it only after you've thoroughly wet your skin in the shower. Using your hands, a loofah, or a washcloth, rub the mixture all over your body (but not on the face), using slow, circular movements, from your extremities toward your torso. Be sure to rinse off completely.

· Try an oatmeal bath (you'll find a recipe in the following pages) or soak in Kneipp Almond Blossom Moisture Bath ($17) for a moisturizing treatment. Sweet almond oil contains vitamins and minerals that are beneficial to the skin and very gentle.

· Don't dry off with a towel—it will rob your skin of much-needed moisture. Instead apply body oil while still in the tub, and then put on a terry robe. Once you've brushed your teeth, applied facial moisturizer, and so on, your skin will be dry enough to pat gently with a towel.

· Don't skip the body oil; not only is it great for feeling pampered, but it also helps your skin retain moisture as it dries. Body oil is best applied while skin is still slightly damp. Johnson's Baby Oil ($3.80), with aloe vera, is an old favorite, but you can also try Burt's Bees Apricot Baby Oil ($14), part of Burt's all-natural Baby Bee collection. This product keeps skin nicely moisturized, and its smell is indescribable. An added benefit: It works great as a light hair oil.

Do-It-Yourself Skin Care

Try these cheap and oh-so-simple concoctions to ease dry skin:

Oatmeal Scrub for Your Face

1. Mix regular rolled oats—not instant oats—with enough milk to make a paste.
2. Let the mixture sit for a few minutes, until the oats start to plump a little.

3. Use gently as a face scrub, making sure you rinse well.

Salt Scrub for Your Body

1. Use a base oil of jojoba, macadamia, hazelnut, or olive oil.
2. Add enough table or kosher salt to the oil to make a paste.
3. Use as a body scrub, but be sure *not* to use a salt scrub right after shaving. Ouch!

Oatmeal Bath

1. If your entire body is feeling parched, put 1/2 to 1 cup of old-fashioned rolled oats into a muslin bag or handkerchief.
2. Close securely with a rubber band.
3. Place the bag in the tub and run warm water.

32

FACE FORWARD:

Simple Fixes
for **Fabulous Skin**

You own an arsenal of skin-care products and religiously follow the instructions to the letter. Yet your skin still seems to be lacking that special glow. But by improving your skin awareness and making just a few small changes in your lifestyle and beauty regimen, you can achieve the often elusive goal of clear, radiant skin.

The first question to ask, and answer: What's your type?

Know Your Skin

Any skin-care routine is less likely to work if you begin it without knowing your skin type. Too often, women with sensitive skin unwittingly use harsh products, or ladies who are prone to oiliness overmoisturize.

The four skin types are dry, normal or combination, oily, and sensitive. To determine which one best describes you, try this simple test:

Wash your face as you normally would, but do not apply

moisturizer. Wait 15 minutes and then take a white tissue and lightly press it to your skin. If the tissue sticks to your skin or becomes translucent in many areas, your skin is oily. If the tissue is clean when you remove it, your skin is dry.

Oiliness in the T-zone (forehead, nose, and chin) means normal or combination skin. Although sensitive skin cannot be determined from this test, that label probably applies if you are prone to minor breakouts or irritations from products or the wind and sun. Regardless of skin type or tone, we all—even black folks—need a daily sunscreen of at least SPF 15, year-round, to protect our skin from the potentially cancerous effects of the sun's ultraviolet radiation.

Clean It Up

Yes, of course you wash your face, but are you cleaning it *correctly*? Some dos and don'ts to remember:

1. Consider switching to a gentle facial cleanser rather than regular soap, which is basically a detergent that is usually too harsh for facial skin.
2. Wash in the morning and at night to remove makeup, pollution, dirt, and the dead skin cells that can dull your complexion.
3. Never go to bed wearing makeup, which can cause clogged pores and breakouts (not to mention messy pillowcases).
4. Always follow washing with a moisturizer suited to your skin type.

Watch Your Mouth

What you eat and drink has a direct effect on the condition of your skin. The foundation of a skin-friendly diet is drinking at least 8 8-ounce glasses of water a day. Fruits, vegetables, and most fiber-rich foods will also help keep you hydrated and rid your skin of toxins. A diet lacking in fatty acids (from foods such as nuts and avocados) can cause skin to lose its luster, while one rich in antioxidants (from leafy green and yellow vegetables) will guarantee a glow.

Cigarettes are one of the worst things you can put in your mouth, not only for health but also for aesthetic reasons. Smoking reduces oxygen to the skin, which slows down the formation of the collagen that is crucial to skin's elasticity and suppleness.

For More Beauty Buzz...

Check out these two books for more tips on beautifying your skin:

Brown Skin: Dr. Susan Taylor's Prescription for Flawless Skin, Hair, and Nails by Susan C. Taylor, M.D. ($14.95; HarperCollins).

Beautiful Skin of Color by Jeanine Downie, M.D., and Fran Cook-Bolden, M.D., with Barbara Nevins Taylor ($25.95; HarperCollins).

33

TEN STEPS TO

Healthier Hair

One of Whoopi Goldberg's most memorable career moments came when she put a towel on her head and pretended to be a little girl yearning for hair that would flow down her back. It struck a chord because at some time or another, many black women have been that girl—and for some of us, the desire for back-skimming hair has been lifelong.

Although it is not self-affirming to chase a beauty image that may be unattainable, it is a worthwhile goal to strive for hair that is at its most glorious and healthy. And as Linda Amerson, Ph.D.—a Dallas-based trichologist who specializes in African American hair loss and scalp disorders—explains, we may be sabotaging our own efforts to grow our hair by embracing harmful styling techniques and lifestyle choices. Here, Dr. Amerson lays down the facts to help your hair live up (or down) to its potential.

8 Barriers Between You and Longer Hair

Genetics. "Not everyone is predisposed to have long hair," says Dr. Amerson. It is DNA—the nucleic acid formulas in cells—that determines much about hair's length, density, and texture. That said, everyone can achieve a healthy mane, provided she takes heed of the other culprits. . .

Chemicals. "Chemical alopecia, which leads to scalp damage, is the most common reason black women's hair does not grow," our expert warns. Caused by years of using relaxers, dye, and other harsh products, this condition can lead to infections and inflammation as well as stunted hair growth. Tip: Allow two months between relaxer touch-ups, and never break the cardinal rule of waiting at least 14 days between a relaxer treatment and a coloring treatment.

Weaves and braids. The styles themselves are not the problem, but too often they are put in too tightly, leading to a condition called traction alopecia, which can damage hair follicles and cause them to atrophy. Ask your hairstylist to ease up on the tension, even if it means your style will not last as long.

Dr. Amerson also cautions against overzealous twisting of new growth, which can cause breakage at the hairline for lock wearers. Tip: Stimulate your scalp to improve blood circulation to your hair follicles. Each night, take your fingertips and knead for 5 to 10 minutes.

What you eat. "Healthy hair and scalp need a nutritious diet," stresses Dr. Amerson. This includes proper nutrients, carbohydrates, and sufficient water, all of which may be lacking in the fast-paced lifestyles and crash diets to which many women subject themselves. Tip: Dr. Amerson says that vitamin and mineral supplements are helpful. She recommends taking B complex, C, A, and folic acid supplements.

Your health. Certain health conditions, such as diabetes, anemia, and thyroid problems, can affect the rate of your hair growth, as can using oral contraceptives or high blood pressure medication. Hormonal changes, whether from your menstrual cycle, hormone replacement therapy, or other reasons, can also be a factor. So if you see a sudden change in hair-shedding or hair-growth patterns, get a complete checkup to determine if there's a medical reason.

The elements. Yes, sun feels good on your face and gives your (SPF-covered) skin such a wonderful glow. But according to Dr. Amerson, the ultraviolet rays can cause considerable damage to your hair and scalp. "And both sun and the wind can cause extensive dryness," she adds. Blustery conditions can cause more than just bad hair days; constant exposure to strong winds can actually cause split ends.

Tip: Use hats and scarves to cover up at the beach and to shield your hair on windy days. Or protect hair and scalp with products containing shea butter, a natural sunscreen. Try Hamadi Shea Hair Cream ($23 for 4 oz.), an excellent choice whether your hair is straight, natural, braided, or in locks.

How you handle your hair. "Black textured hair is extremely vulnerable because our hair grows, curls, and loops around other hair shafts, which leads to knotting, breaking, and tangled hair," Dr. Amerson explains. Wear a silk scarf at night, or drape one over your pillow, to avoid breakage caused by friction. Take time when detangling wet hair, and always use a wide-toothed comb, a good conditioner, and a gentle hand.

Try Carol's Daughter Khoret Amen Shea Butter Hair Smoothie conditioner ($10).

How often you trim it. "Cutting on a regular basis does help considerably because then your hair is not splitting up the shaft," says Dr. Amerson. Although it may sound counterintuitive, losing an inch or two every so often will actually result in longer, healthier hair. That's why you should be going in for trims every six weeks.

And 2 Factors That Make No Difference

The seasons. Contrary to what many people insist, Dr. Amerson says, there is no scientific evidence that hair grows faster in the summer. "What may account for that belief is that when it's hot outside, some people don't use as much heat in their hair, meaning there's not as high a chance of damage." Tip: If you decide to let your hair dry naturally, invest in a good leave-in conditioner, such as that from Bumble and Bumble ($24.99), to fight frizz and keep hair moisturized.

Hair-growth pills, creams, and lotions. "I am of the opinion that most of these products are not the answer," says Dr. Amerson. Although some people see positive results with minoxidil, a prescription solution that stimulates growth, she stresses that "you must know what type of alopecia or scalp disorder you have before you try to fix it."

RESOURCE GUIDE

GENERAL HEALTH

Black Women's Health Imperative

Description: The National Black Women's Health Imperative is a leading African American health education, research, advocacy, and leadership development institution.

Email: nbwhp@nbwhp.org

Address: 600 Pennsylvania Avenue, S.E., Suite 310,
         Washington, D.C. 20003

Phone: (202) 548-4000

Fax: (202) 543-9743

Web: http://www.blackwomenshealth.org

National Women's Health Information Center

Description: This government website and toll-free call center were created to provide free, reliable health information for American women. The website includes a Minority Women's Health section (http://www.4woman.gov/minority/index.htm).

Phone: (800) 994-WOMAN (9662)

Web: http://www.4woman.gov/index.htm

The National Medical Association (NMA)

Description: NMA is the largest and oldest national organization representing African American physicians and their patients in the United States. The site provides a Physician Referral Service for African American doctors.

Address: Executive Offices, 1012 Tenth Street, N.W.,
        Washington, DC 20001

Phone: (202) 347-1895

Fax: (202) 898-2510

Web: http://www.nmanet.org

Findablackdoctor.com

Description: Started by Harlem-based dermatologist Dr. Dina Strachan, Findablackdoctor.com is a free internet service allowing the public to locate U.S.-based African American physicians, as well as dentists, podiatrists, clinical psychologists, and other health care providers. However, searches for medical professionals beyond the U.S. Northeast and Midwest sometimes come up empty.

Address: 55 W. 116th Street, Suite 334, New York, NY 10026

Phone: (877) 581-9512

Fax: (877) 581-9512

Web: http://www.findablackdoctor.com

FamilyDoctor.org

Description: Sponsored by American Academy of Family Physicians, this resource provides information on various health topics for the whole family.

Address: 11400 Tomahawk Creek Parkway, Leawood, KS 66211-2672

Phone: (800) 274-2237

Email: email@familydoctor.org

Web: http://www.familydoctor.org

ALTERNATIVE MEDICINE AND PRACTITIONERS

American Association of Naturopathic Physicians (AANP)

Description: The AANP provides information and resources about naturopathic medicine and includes a search feature to find naturopathic physicians.

Address: 3201 New Mexico Avenue, N.W., Suite 350,
   Washington, DC 20016

Phone: (866) 538-2267

Fax: (202) 274-1992

Email: member.services@naturopathic.org

Web: http://www.naturopathic.org/

National Center for Complementary and Alternative Medicine (NCCAM)

Description: The NCCAM website includes publications, information for researchers, frequently asked questions, and links to other complementary and alternative-related resources.

Address: NCCAM Clearinghouse, P.O. Box 7923, Gaithersburg, MD 20898

Phone: (888) 644-6226

Fax: (866) 464-3616

E-mail: info@nccam.nih.gov

Web: http://nccam.nih.gov

National Center for Homeopathy

Description: This site provides of information about homeopathy—what it is, research that supports its effectiveness, how you can find a homeopathic practitioner.

Address: 801 N. Fairfax Street, Suite 306, Alexandria, VA 22314

Phone: (703) 548-7790

Fax: (703) 548-7792

Email: info@homeopathic.org

Web: http://www.homeopathic.org

CANCER

National Cancer Institute

Description: The National Cancer Institute coordinates the National
Cancer Program, which conducts and supports research, training,
health information dissemination, and other programs with respect
to the cause, diagnosis, prevention, and treatment of cancer, rehabilitation from cancer, and the continuing care of cancer patients and the
families of cancer patients.
Phone: (800) 4-CANCER (422-6237)
Web: http://www.cancer.gov

American Cancer Society (ACS)

Description: ACS is a nationwide, community-based voluntary health
organization committed to fighting cancer through balanced programs
of research, education, patient service, advocacy, and rehabilitation.
Address: National Home Office, 1559 Clifton Road, NE, Atlanta, GA 30329
Phone: (800) ACS-2345
Web: http://www.cancer.org

Susan G. Komen Breast Cancer Foundation

Description: The Komen Foundation is fighting to eradicate breast can-
cer as a life-threatening disease by funding research grants and sup-
porting education, screening, and treatment projects in communities
around the world.
Address: 5005 LBJ Freeway, Suite 250, Dallas, TX 75244
Phone: (972) 855-1600
Helpline: (800) I'M AWARE
Fax: (972) 855-1605
Web: http://www.komen.org

BreastCancer.org

Description: Breastcancer.org is a nonprofit organization dedicated
to providing the most reliable, complete, and up-to-date information
about breast cancer.
Address: 111 Forrest Avenue, 1R, Narberth, PA 19072
Web: http://www.breastcancer.org

DEPRESSION AND MENTAL HEALTH

National Institute of Mental Health (NIMH)

Description: The NIMH health information center provides information on signs and symptoms, diagnosis, and treatment of various mental health disorders including depression, attention deficit disorders, and anxiety disorders.

Address: Office of Communications, 6001 Executive Boulevard,
Room 8184, MSC 9663, Bethesda, MD 20892-9663

Phone: (866) 615-6464

Fax: (301) 443-4279

Email: nimhinfo@nih.gov

Web: http://www.nimh.nih.gov/healthinformation

National Mental Health Association

Description: The National Mental Health Association is one of the country's oldest and largest nonprofit organizations addressing all aspects of mental health and mental illness. Its website includes fact sheets on mental health issues for people of color, a mental health practitioner locator, and links to local support groups.

Address: 2001 N. Beauregard Street, 12th Floor, Alexandria, VA 22311

Phone: (800) 969-NMHA

Web: http://www.nmha.org

Depression-Screening.org

Description: Sponsored by the National Mental Health Association (NMHA), this site is designed to educate people about clinical depression, offer a confidential way for people to get screened for symptoms of the illness, and guide people toward appropriate professional help if necessary.

Address: 2001 N. Beauregard Street, 12th Floor, Alexandria, Virginia 22311

Phone: (800) 969-NMHA

Fax: (703) 684-5968

Web: http://www.depression-screening.org

DIABETES

The American Diabetes Association

Description: The American Diabetes Association is the nation's leading nonprofit health organization providing diabetes research, information and advocacy.

Address: National Call Center, 1701 N. Beauregard Street,
        Alexandria, VA 22311

Phone: (800) DIABETES (342-2383)

Email: AskADA@diabetes.org

Web: http://www.diabetes.org

Blackandbrownsugar.com

Description: This site was created to provide accurate information to both healthcare professionals and people with diabetes regarding the care and management of diabetes in minority populations.

Address: Black & Brown Sugar, Inc., 310 E. Florence Ave,
        Inglewood, CA 90301

Phone: (626) 798-8819

Fax: (626) 791-9856

Email: info@blackandbrownsugar.com

Web: http://www.blackandbrownsugar.com

FIBROIDS

Medline Plus: Uterine Fibroids

Description: Provided by the U.S. National Library of Medicine, this resource offers information on fibroids, their effects, and various forms of treatment.

Address: U.S. National Library of Medicine, 8600 Rockville Pike,
        Bethesda, MD 20894

Phone: (888) 346-3656

Fax: (301) 402-1384

Email: custserv@nlm.nih.gov

Web: http://www.nlm.nih.gov/medlineplus/uterinefibroids.html

HEALTH AND FITNESS

Health Club Locator

Description: Provided by the American Council on Exercise, this is a
handy resource to find a health club in your area.
Address: 4851 Paramount Drive, San Diego, CA 92123
Phone: (800) 825-3636
Web: http://www.acefitness.org/clublocator

Voice of Dance

Description: Sponsored by Danskin, this website provides information
on finding local dance lessons and has a global directory of over 25,000
dance-related companies and organizations. Use it to find classes in
African and Brazilian-style dancing, Capoeira, jazz movement, salsa,
and more.
Address: 850 College Avenue, Kentfield, CA 94904
Phone: (415) 460-5150
Email: info@voiceofdance.com
Web: http://www.voiceofdance.com/Classes/ClassMain.cfm

The International Association of Black Yoga Teachers (IABYT)

Description: The IABYT is an organization dedicated to increasing the
presence of yoga in the inner city. The site features a search function
to locate black yoga teachers in your area.
Address: P.O. Box 360922, Los Angeles, CA 90036
Phone: (213) 833-6371
Email: yoga@blackyogateachers.com
Web: http://www.blackyogateachers.com

YogaFinder.com

Description: The largest yoga directory on the internet, including
worldwide locations and information on teacher's training, retreats,
yoga workshops, yoga conferences.
Email: webmaster@yogafinder.com
Web: http://www.yogafinder.com

YMCA of the USA

Description: The YMCA provides resources and activities in local communities to foster strong kids, strong families, and strong communities.
Address: 101 N. Wacker Drive, Chicago, IL 60606
Phone: (312) 977-0031
Web: http://www.ymca.net

HEALTHY DIET

Interactive Menu Planner

Description: Created by the National Heart, Lung, and Blood Institute, this interactive menu planner is designed to guide daily food and meal choices based on one day's calorie allowance. It may be used in advance to plan a meal or at the end of a day to add up total calories, fat, and carbohydrates consumed.
Address: NHLBI Health Information Center, P.O. Box 30105,
Bethesda, MD 20824-0105
Phone: (301) 592-8573
Email: nhlbiinfo@nhlbi.nih.gov
Web: http://hin.nhlbi.nih.gov/menuplanner

MedlinePlus Drinking Water Resource Page

Description: Provided by the U.S. National Library of Medicine, this resource provides information on the importance of water in a healthy diet.
Address: U.S. National Library of Medicine, 8600 Rockville Pike,
Bethesda, MD 20894
Phone: (888) 346-3656
Fax: (301) 402-1384
Email: custserv@nlm.nih.gov
Web: http://www.nlm.nih.gov/medlineplus/drinkingwater.html

U.S. Department of Agriculture National Organic Program

Description: The National Organic Program provides consumers with information on organic food standards and is a great resource for those looking to increase the amount of organic foods in their diet.

Address: Room 4008-South Building, 1400 Independence Avenue, S.W.,
        Washington, DC 20250-0020

Phone: (202) 720-3252

Fax: (202) 205-7808

Web: http://www.ams.usda.gov/nop/indexIE.htm

HEART AND STROKE

The National Coalition for Women With Heart Disease

Description: Learn about the unique symptoms, treatments, and challenges experienced by women with heart disease through this nonprofit coalition of health organizations, which is also known as WomenHeart.

Address: 818 18th Street, N.W., Suite 230, Washington, DC 20006

Phone: (202) 728-7199

Web: http://www.womenheart.org

American Heart Association (AHA)

Description: The AHA provides information on reducing your chances of disability and death from cardiovascular diseases and stroke.

Address: National Center, 7272 Greenville Avenue, Dallas, TX 75231

Phone: (800) AHA-USA-1

Web: http://www.americanheart.org

American Stroke Association (ASA)

Description: The ASA is the division of the American Heart Association that provides information on avoiding disability and death from stroke through research, education, fund raising, and advocacy.

Address: National Center, 7272 Greenville Avenue, Dallas, TX 75231

Phone: (888) 4-STROKE

Web: http://www.strokeassociation.org

PREGNANCY AND FERTILITY

iVillage Pregnancy and Parenting
Description: From trying to conceive through your child's teen years, iVillage Pregnancy & Parenting offers up-to-date and informative articles, features, and expert advice.
Web: http://parenting.ivillage.com

The American Fertility Association (AFA)
Description: The AFA's purpose is to educate the public about reproductive disease and support families during their struggles with infertility and adoption.
Address: 666 Fifth Avenue, Suite 278, New York, NY 10103
Phone: (888) 917-3777
Fax: (718) 601-7722
E-mail: info@theafa.org
Web: http://www.theafa.org

The National Infertility Association (RESOLVE)
Description: The mission of RESOLVE is to provide timely, compassionate support and information to people who are experiencing infertility and to increase awareness of infertility issues through public education and advocacy.
Address: 7910 Woodmont Avenue, Suite 1350, Bethesda, MD 20814
Phone: (301) 652-8585
Fax: (301) 652-9375
Email: info@resolve.org
Web: http://www.resolve.org

SEXUAL HEALTH

American Social Health Association (ASHA)
Description: ASHA is recognized by the public, patients, providers, and policymakers for developing and delivering accurate, medically reliable information about STDs.
Address: P.O. Box 13827, Research Triangle Park, NC 27709
Phone: (919) 361-8400
Fax: (919) 361-8425
Web: http://www.ashastd.org

Black AIDS Institute
Description: Learn about HIV prevention, AIDS treatment, rising infection rates among black women, and the especially devastating effects of this epidemic on the black community.
Address: 1833 W. 8th Street, Suite 200, Los Angeles, CA 90057
Phone: (213) 353-3610
Web: http://www.blackaids.org

Planned Parenthood Federation of America, Inc.
Description: Planned Parenthood–affiliated health centers nationwide provide high quality, affordable reproductive health care and sexual health information for women, men, and teens.
Address: 434 W. 33rd Street, New York, NY 10001
Phone: (800) 230-PLAN
Web: http://www.plannedparenthood.com

SKIN PROBLEMS

National Eczema Association for Science and Education (NEASE)

Description: NEASE works to improve the health and the quality of life of all persons living with atopic dermatitis/eczema, providing emotional support, information, and resources to those who have the disease as well as their loved ones, while raising public awareness of the disease.

Address: 4460 Redwood Highway, Suite 16-D, San Rafael, CA 94903-1953

Phone: (800) 818-7546

Fax: (415) 472-5345

Email: info@nationaleczema.org

Web: http://www.nationaleczema.org/home.html

American Academy of Dermatology: Find a Dermatologist

Description: This resource provides detailed biographical informa-tion about academy-member dermatologists who participate in their Profile Program, including information about their education, special-ized training, office hours, healthcare plan participation, and more.

Address: 1350 I Street, N.W., Suite 870, Washington, DC 20005-4355

Phone: (888) 462-DERM

Web: http://www.aad.org/public/searchderm.htm

SPA RESOURCES

Spa Finder

Description: Spa Finder is one of the leading spa travel and marketing companies connecting consumers with the spa experience via publish-ing, travel, internet, and corporate incentive services.

Address: 257 Park Avenue S., floor 10, New York, NY 10010

Phone: (212) 924-6800

Web: http://www.spafinder.com

The Day Spa Association

Description: Provides a directory that will guide you to true day spas that meets the guidelines of The Day Spa Association.
Address: 310 17th Street, Union City, NJ 07087
Phone: (201) 865-2065
Email: info@dayspaassociation.com
Web: http://www.dayspaassociation.com/

THYROID DISEASE AND AUTOIMMUNE DISORDERS

American Autoimmune Related Diseases Association

Description: Find out about rheumatoid arthritis, lupus, and other autoimmune diseases affecting women at the AARDA's website.
Address: 22100 Gratiot Avenue, East Detroit, MI 48021
Phone: (586)776-3900
Web: http://www.aarda.org

The American Thyroid Association (ATA)

Description: Get information about thyroid-related diseases via the ATA's patient information FAQs.
Address: 6066 Leesburg Pike, Suite 550, Falls Church, Virginia 22041
Phone: (800) THYROID
Email: admin@thyroid.org
Web: http://www.thyroid.org/patients/patients.html

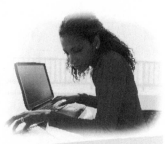 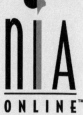
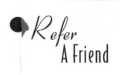